MEMORY GAMES
FOR SENIORS

Memory Boosting Activities for
Overcoming Dementia

by

Blaine R.

Disclaimer Notice

This book has been independently written and published. Kindly note that the content contained within this publication is provided exclusively for informational and entertainment purposes. Every effort has been made to provide accurate, current, reliable, and complete information. No express or implied assurances are present. The content of this book is intended to aid readers in attaining a more comprehensive understanding of the related subject. The exercises, information, and activities are designed exclusively for self-help. This book does not intend to serve as a substitute for the counsel of professional psychologists, attorneys, financiers, or other experts. Kindly contact a certified professional if you need counseling.

Reading this work, the reader agrees that the author shall not be responsible for any direct or indirect harm caused by the content contained herein, including but not restricted to omissions, errors, or inaccuracies. You are responsible for the decisions, actions, and outcomes that ensue as a reader.

About the Author

Blaine R. is an experienced professional in cognitive therapy for all ages; notably, he enjoys assisting seniors. With extensive knowledge and practical experience, he is a speaker and author on mental health. His passion for comforting dementia in seniors by encouraging them in unconventional ways like playing games, conversations and solving challenging memory games makes him to write a book especially for them to enhance their emotional resilience, improve memory, and promote healthy social and communication skills. His work has helped countless seniors overcome emotional and memory challenges, developing them into confident and resilient individuals.

Table of Content

A Special Note

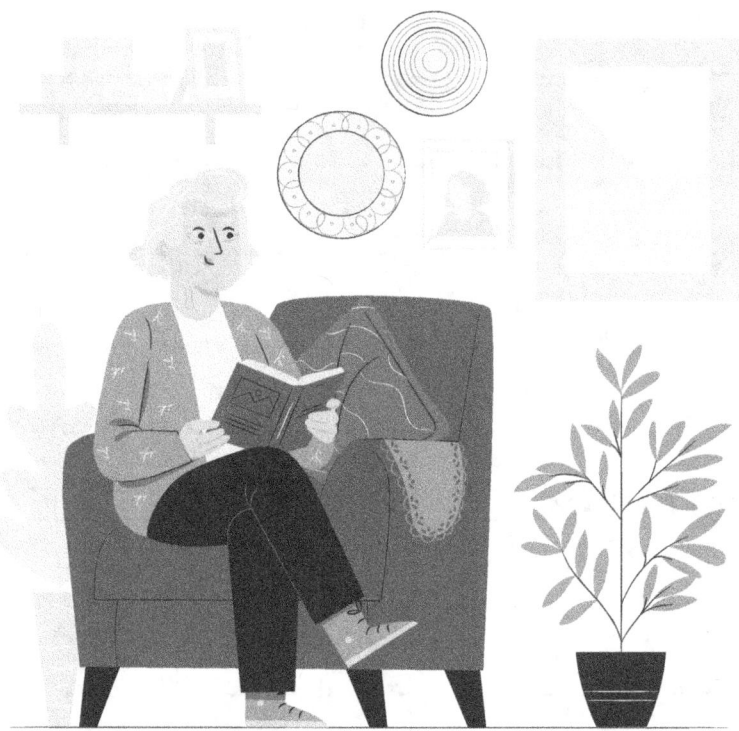

As you age, changes occur in all of your body parts, including the brain. As a result, some of you notice that you don't remember details about the surroundings and past, and even after continuous trying, you still feel unable to recall them quickly. You may sometimes need to be corrected to remember names and home addresses. By keeping your challenges in mind, we have designed a memory book that comprises of information about dementia and, most importantly, several brain games that are specially tailored to meet your requirements. These games intend to improve your brain's cognitive functioning and retain memory. This book is an effective source to keep you engaged and busy, simultaneously improving your mental health. So, without wasting time, let's explore this resource.

Introduction: Dementia- At a Glance

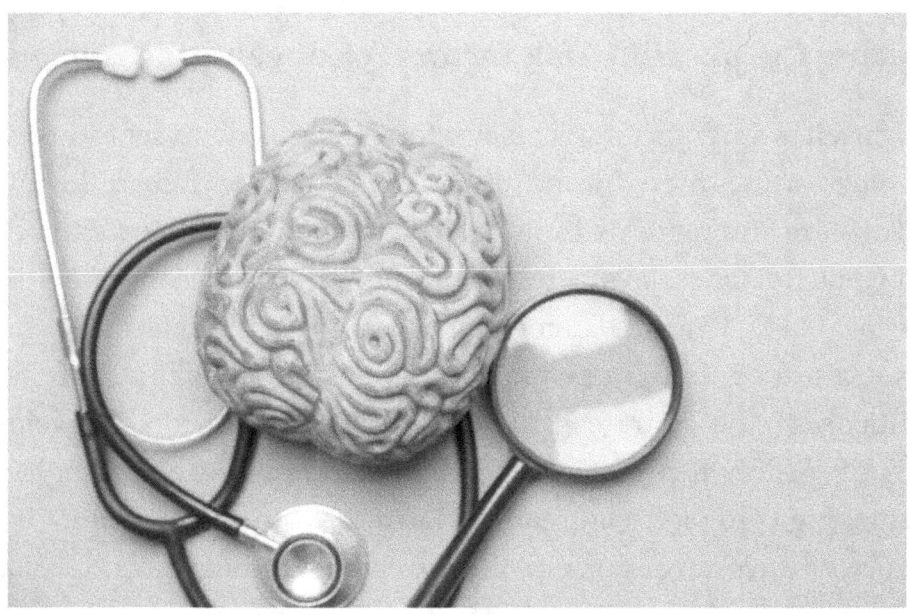

Dementia is not a typical disease but a general term for the inability to recall, think, or make findings that meddle with day-to-day activities. Alzheimer's disease is the most typical sort of dementia. Though dementia primarily impacts older adults, it is not a part of standard aging.

Symptoms of dementia

The symptoms of dementia may vary widely from person to person due to the vast nature of the term. Dementia is an illness that can cause tribulations with multiple cognitive functions, like memory, concentration, communication, logic, assessment, problem-solving, and visual perception, further the regular age-related differences in vision. Some signs that may

Aging is a natural process that affects our physical and mental capacities and can raise disease risk. According to the WHO, its effect varies from person to person, and healthy aging is a fundamental right of every human being.

signify dementia are getting lost in familiar places, utilizing unusual words for familiar entities, forgetting the names of dear friends or relatives, forgetting old memories, and having problems finishing tasks independently.

What are the possible risk factors for developing dementia?

Aging itself is a significant risk factor for dementia, with seniors 65 years and older being more prone to it. Those with a family history of dementia are also more susceptible to developing the illness. Ethnicity is another factor that plays a role, with aged African Americans living twice as likely to catch dementia as compared to whites, whereas Hispanics are 1.5 times more likely to suffer from dementia. Poor health conditions of the heart can also increase the chance of developing dementia, mainly if conditions like high blood pressure and cholesterol or smoking are left untreated. Further, traumatic brain injury, specifically if it's severe or repetitious, can raise the risk of developing dementia.

What are the most common types of dementia?

Dementia is a cluster of symptoms that usually affect memory, thinking, and social abilities. Different diseases and health conditions can provoke it, some of which are reversible. Nonetheless, the most familiar types of dementia are:

- ✓ Alzheimer's disease

- ✓ Vascular dementia

- ✓ Lewy body dementia

- ✓ Frontotemporal dementia

- ✓ Mixed dementia

To decrease the probability of developing chronic diseases such as dementia, it is vital to lead a healthy lifestyle by exercising regularly, eating healthy and keeping social connections. Playing memory games or participating in mentally stimulating activities may improve cognitive function and help with memory loss. Living with dementia can be demanding because cognitive tribulations may emerge, like issues with memory, thinking process, logic and reasoning, and speech disorder. Yet, innovative treatment methods can help eliminate these symptoms while nurturing the brain and keeping it busy. Games, in particular, can unite individuals, making them bond perfectly with others and form new memories with loved ones.

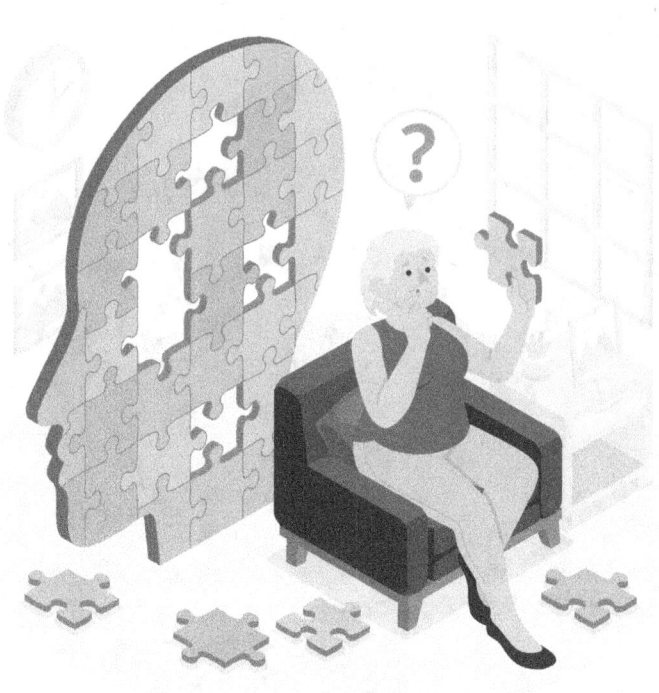

My lovely seniors, the following poster shows four healthy tips to remain mentally fit.

Quick Tips to Retain Memory

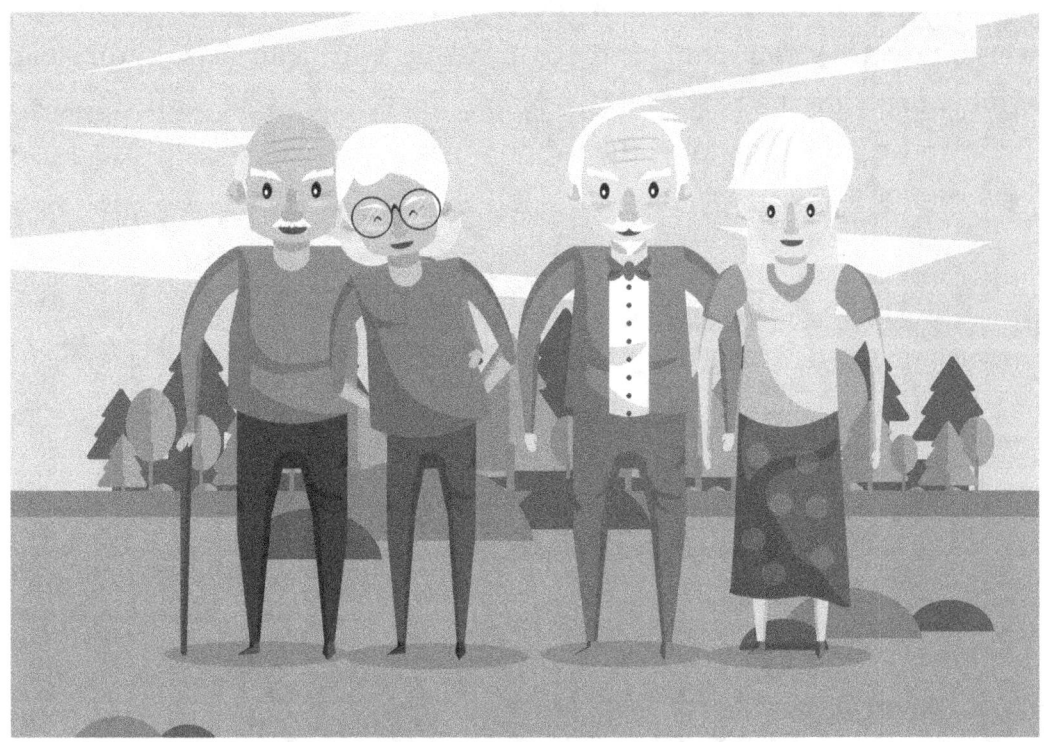

- Be positive

- Eat healthy

- To age well, you need to live well

- Retain memory through brain exercise

My dear seniors, we know memory is something we make every day, and we keep creating fresh ones, but there is something extremely gratifying about rethinking those from a long time ago. For those of you who are suffering from dementia, with a lowered ability to retain short-term memories, it is more critical to recall long-term memories. We have compiled interesting, exciting and colorful activities for you to boost memory retention in this book. There is a separate section for bonus brain games in every chapter. You will find several exercises to enhance cognitive functioning, coordination, and vision. So let's see, what are those bonus brain activities?

Bonus Brain Games

In this book, we have arranged a collection of brain games related to creative, sensory, social connection and memory activities for you to cope with dementia. These resources are specifically designed to enhance your memory and improve cognitive impairment.

◈ Picture Match and Coloring

In this activity, you will have two sets of images related to each other. You need to match them. Coloring is fun for everyone. All you have to do is grab some colors and color the exciting worksheets.

◈ Trivia

A trivia game is designed to ask questions about exciting facts of various interests.

◈ Visual Puzzles

In this activity, you need to analyze two pictures and identify the items present in the first picture and missing in the second picture.

❖ Brain Teasers

Dear seniors, brain teasers such as finding alphabets, constructing words and mazes are the perfect way to activate your brain. They mentally engage you and boost your thinking skills.

❖ Crossword

Crossword is one of the best memory booster games. It helps you retain memory by looking at the picture and writing the correct name of the object.

❖ Word Puzzles

Word puzzles help you increase your vocabulary and activates the brain's cognitive function, which helps to retain memory.

❖ Sudoku

Sudoku is a mind-blowing game for concentration and calculation. It involves a series of numbers in rows and columns.

❖ Pattern Recognition

Pattern recognition is another element of memory games in which you must find the perfect fit for different patterns.

❖ Word Association Chain

In this activity, you need to find the perfect word that has some connection with the previous word.

❖ Scramble Words

In the scramble words activity, you need to look at the image carefully in the worksheet and solve the scrambled words.

◈ Find the Difference

"Find the Difference" worksheets are designed to test your vision and focus.

◈ Counting: How Many

Counting worksheets are an excellent way to help you revise the counting task and retain memory.

◈ Visual Perception

Visual perception worksheets help reduce visual discrimination and improve perceptual and memory skills.

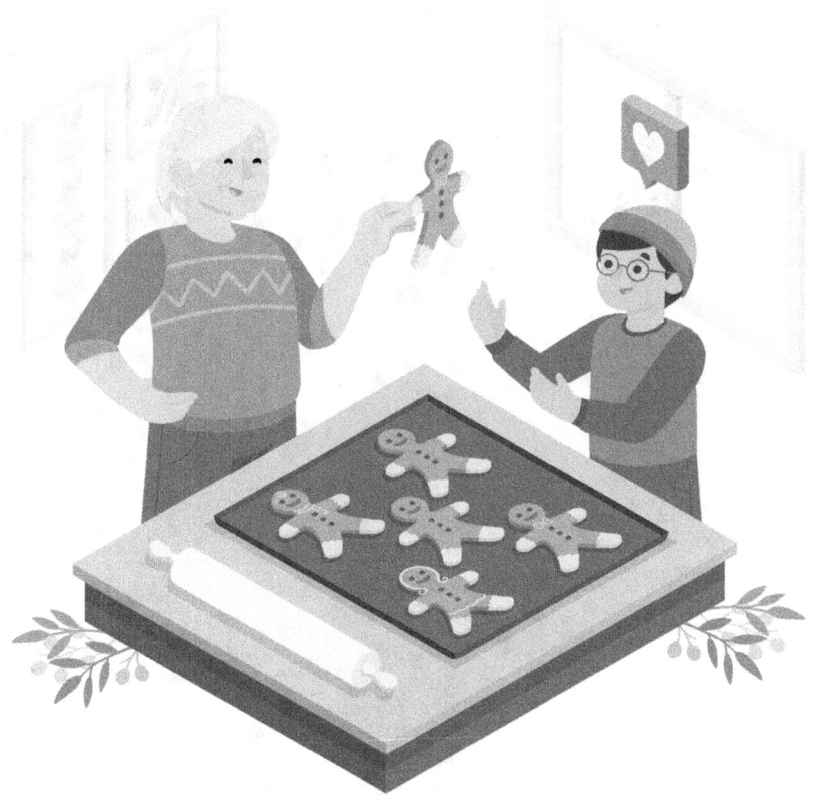

Before moving to the next chapter, mention your top 5 memories in this memory tree:

MY MEMORY TREE

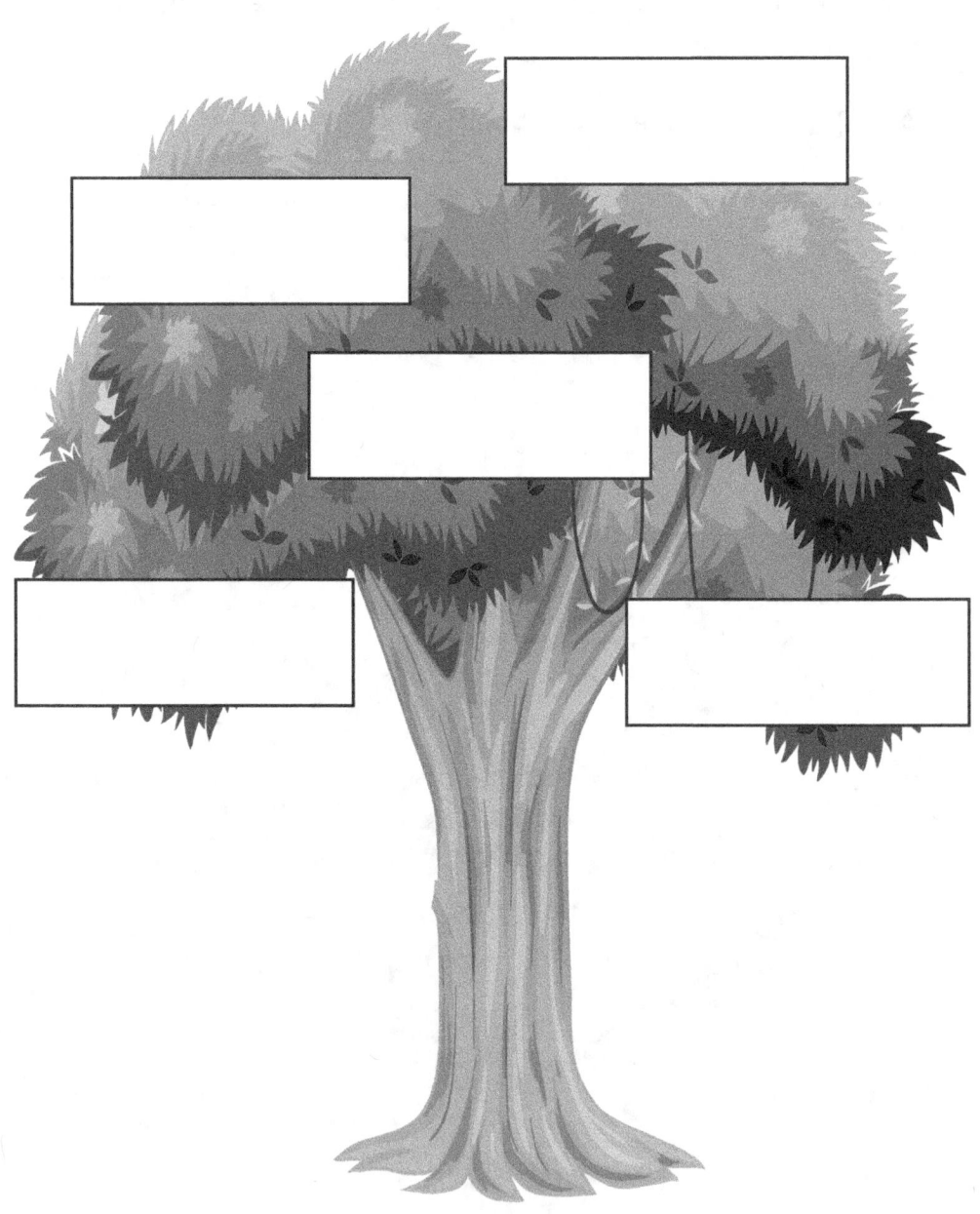

Memory-Boosting Activities at Home - Overcoming Dementia

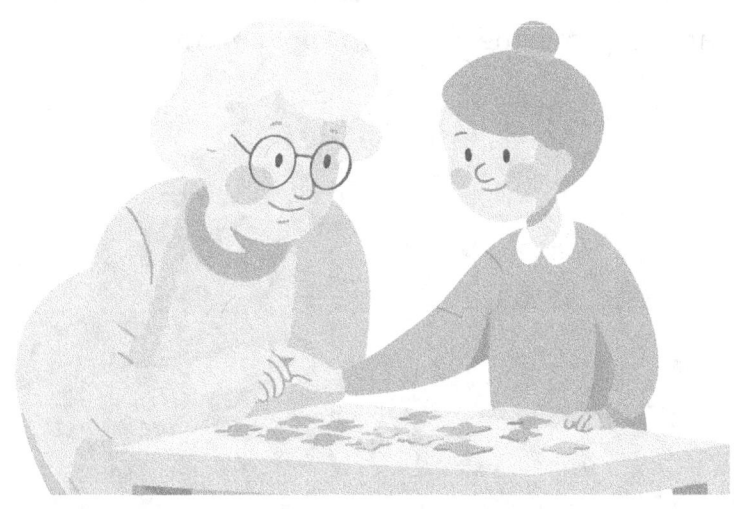

My mother is suffering from dementia, but otherwise she is healthy. I spend time with her, take her on nature walks and hikes, and do mental exercises like coloring, assembling puzzles, and other memory-boosting games to keep her busy and active. I have observed that memory games are crucial as they slow the disease's progression and keep her mind functional. She also enjoys playing memory games; seeing her entertained and having fun is amusing for me. I take photos of our quality time and activities for her to relish later. I admire what she did for me as a kid; now it's my turn to give back to her. Catching her laugh and smile makes me feel close to her again.

(Story of Loretta)

Memory games can benefit you as they can help foster and challenge your brain. Like other body muscles, the brain requires exercise to function properly. The mind-fostering games can support the function of brain cells and even stimulate the growth of fresh ones.

It has been found that playing brain games can improve brain health in people with early and middle-stage dementia, comprising short-term memory, reaction time, socializing, problem-solving, logical reasoning, and communication. Further, memory games help critical thinking and originality while promoting concentration on detail. They uplift visual recognition and improve the ability to spot contrasts.

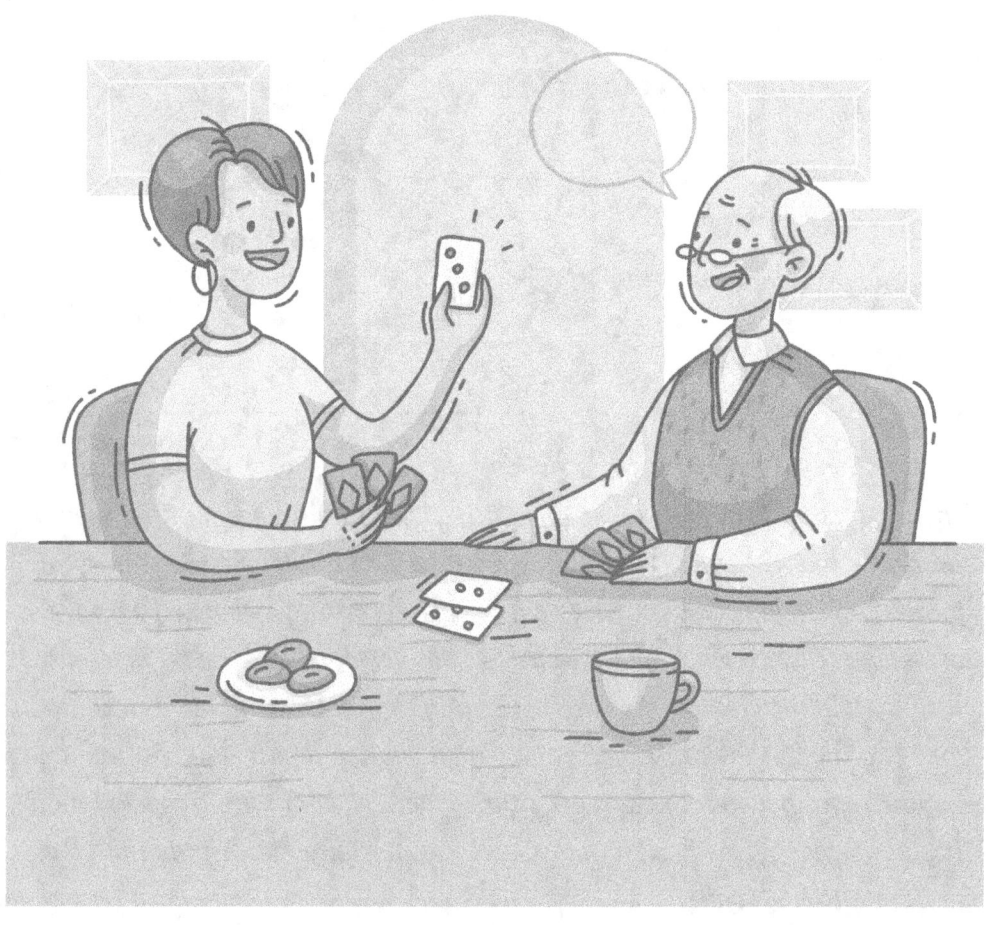

The Box of Memories

Dear seniors, before further exploring memory games, kindly write down some memories of a person you miss.

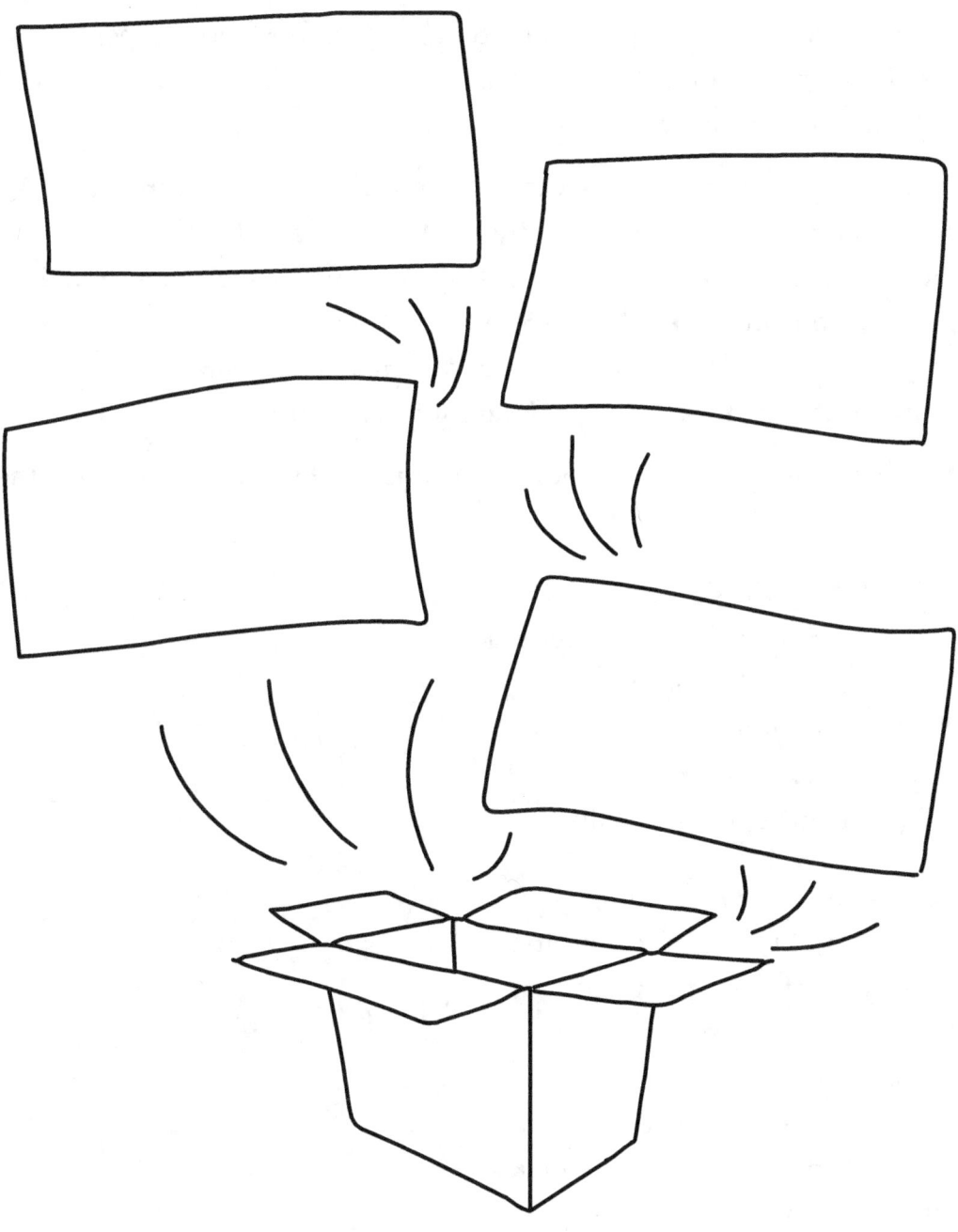

Playing games can also play an incredible role in social interaction and bonding. A friendly competition combined with casual conversation is a helpful way to promote togetherness. As people age, they need more company than youngsters do.

Adopting physical activities can also be beneficial for you. These games can help you improve your balance, coordination, and temper. These activities can be adjusted for various activity levels and can be played indoors and outdoors.

Seniors, it's essential to discover engaging activities tailored to your requirements. What one may find attractive, another may consider mundane. Therefore, sharing with your loved ones is essential to identify your interests. When choosing activities for yourself, consider that they are structured, sensorial, and personalized. There are multiple activities to pick from when looking for activity options.

Yet, when scheduling appropriate activities, it's best to consider the following:

- Your physical constraints
- Individual vs group activities
- Your daily routine
- Your motivation
- Your attractions
- Your functional skills

Cognitive activities for you should concentrate on creativity, sensory stimulants, making social connections, and memory enhancement. It's worth noting that attention deviates from person to person and it may look different to different people.

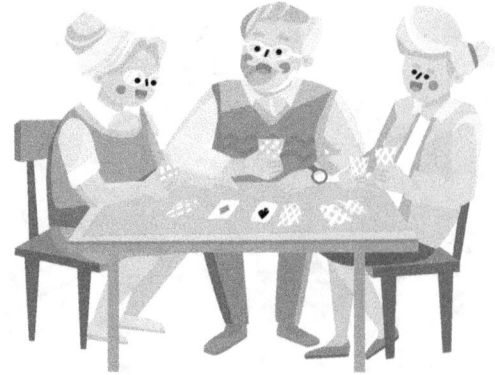

Part - I
1. Creative Activities for Seniors Coping with Dementia

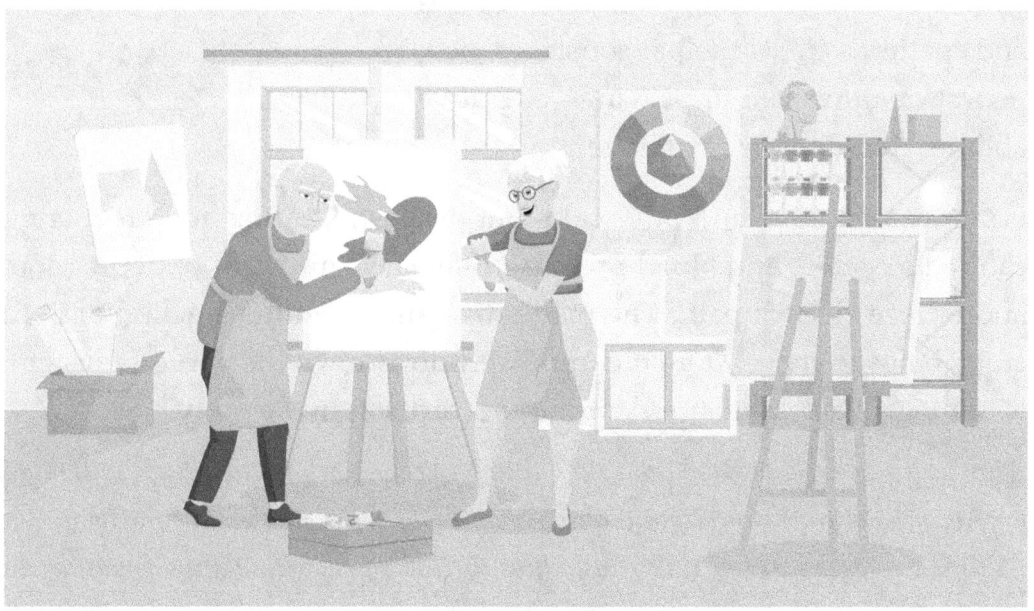

Participating in ventures you excel at is vital, as completing something is a great motivation. This is especially true for you with dementia, for which creative exercises can be the most delightful. Engaging in creative and fulfilling activities can help relieve common dementia symptoms like anxiety, agitation, depression, and anger.

1.1. Knitting or Crocheting

Knitting and crocheting are excellent and productive hobbies for you due to their simple yet complex nature. Both techniques only require sticks and string, but the endless possibilities of combined stitches make them complex.

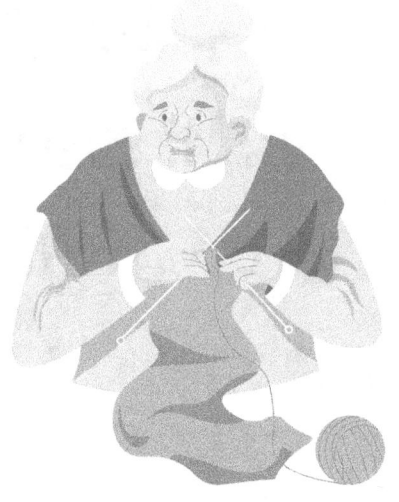

In terms of physical benefits, both knitting and crochet can challenge and support your brain by repeating complex stitches and patterns. This helps construct new neural pathways, improving cognitive abilities that diminish with age.

From the cognitive and physical point of view, knitting and crocheting can reduce stress and blood pressure, alleviate symptoms of depression, and relieve chronic pain. The meditative and repetitious action of both crafts helps to concentrate the mind and slow down the nervous system, lessening anxiety and stress hormones (cortisol) in the body.

Knitting and crochet have been shown to boost memory for dementia patients. According to an investigation by Yonas Geda, a psychiatrist at the Mayo Clinic, engaging in knitting can reduce the risk of cognitive impairment and memory loss in later life.

Thus, knitting and crochet have both the physical and mental health advantages and can enhance the quality of life for those with dementia.

Before going further, let me explain the difference between knitting and crochet. Knitting uses two long needles to create the loops, shifting a batch of loops from one needle to another; the stitches are kept on the needle. Crochet is done using a single hook, to hook the loops directly on the piece. This significant difference makes crochet much more effortless to work with than knitting.

Knitting VS. Crochet

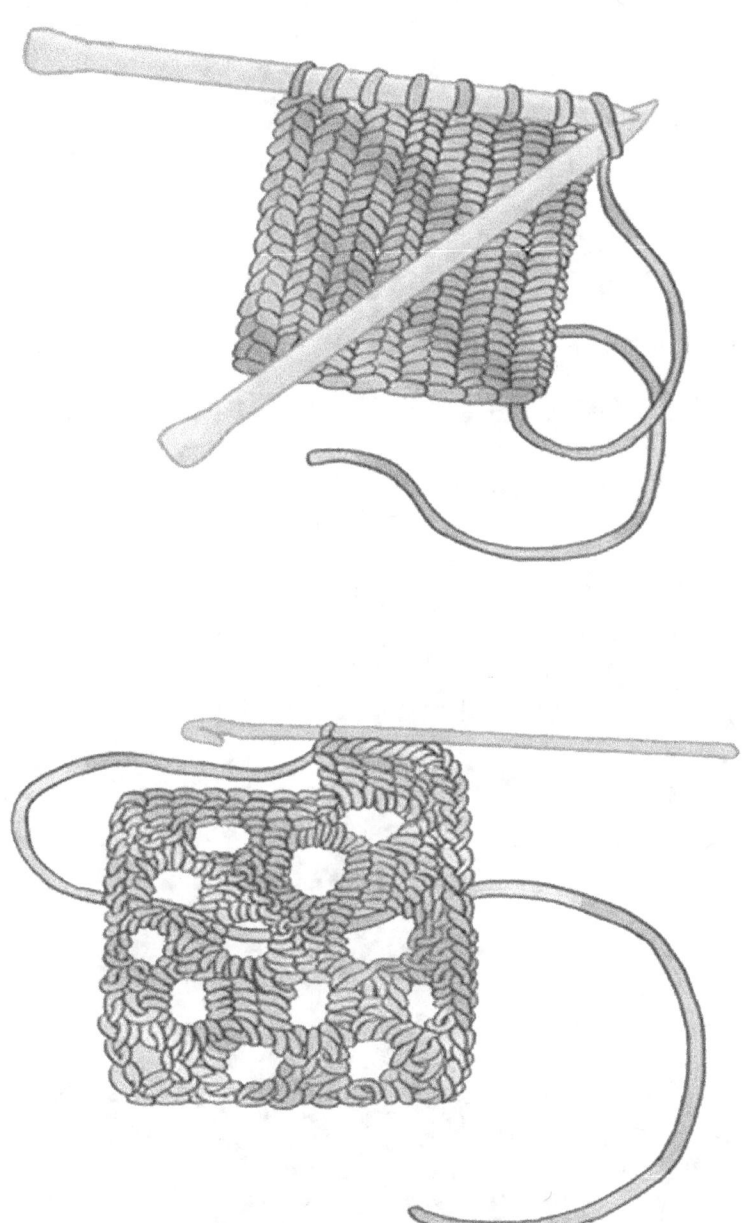

Basic Symbols

The following worksheet guides you about the basic stitches in knitting.

Symbol	Abbr.	Description
○	**Yo**	Yarn over
\	**Ssk**	Slip slip knit
/	**K2tog**	Knit two stitches together
⋏	**Sssk** / **Sk2p**	Slip slip slip knit / Slip stitch, knit two together pass slipped stitch over
⋏	**K3tog**	Knit three stitches together
⋏	**Sssp**	Slip slip slip purl
⋏	**P3tog**	Purl three stitches together
⋀	**S2kp**	Slip two stitches knitwise, knit one, pass slipped stitches over
⋏	**M1lp**	Make one purlwise left leaning
⋏	**M1rp**	Make one purlwise right leaning

Symbol	Abbr.	Description
□	**K**	Knit
⊡	**P**	Purl
Ω	**K tbl**	Knit through the back loop
Ω	**P tbl**	Purl throught the back loop
೦	**M1**	Make one stitch
೦	**M1p**	Make one purlwise
Y	**M1l**	Make one left
Y	**M1r**	Make one right
V	**Sl wyib**	Slip stitch with yarn in back
V	**Sl wyif**	Slip stich with yarn front

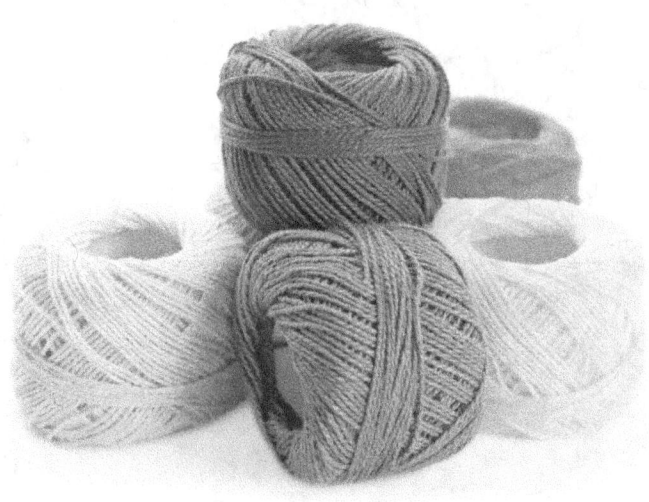

24

The following knitting-themed coloring page can help you create color schemes, improve fine motor skills, and boost cognitive abilities.

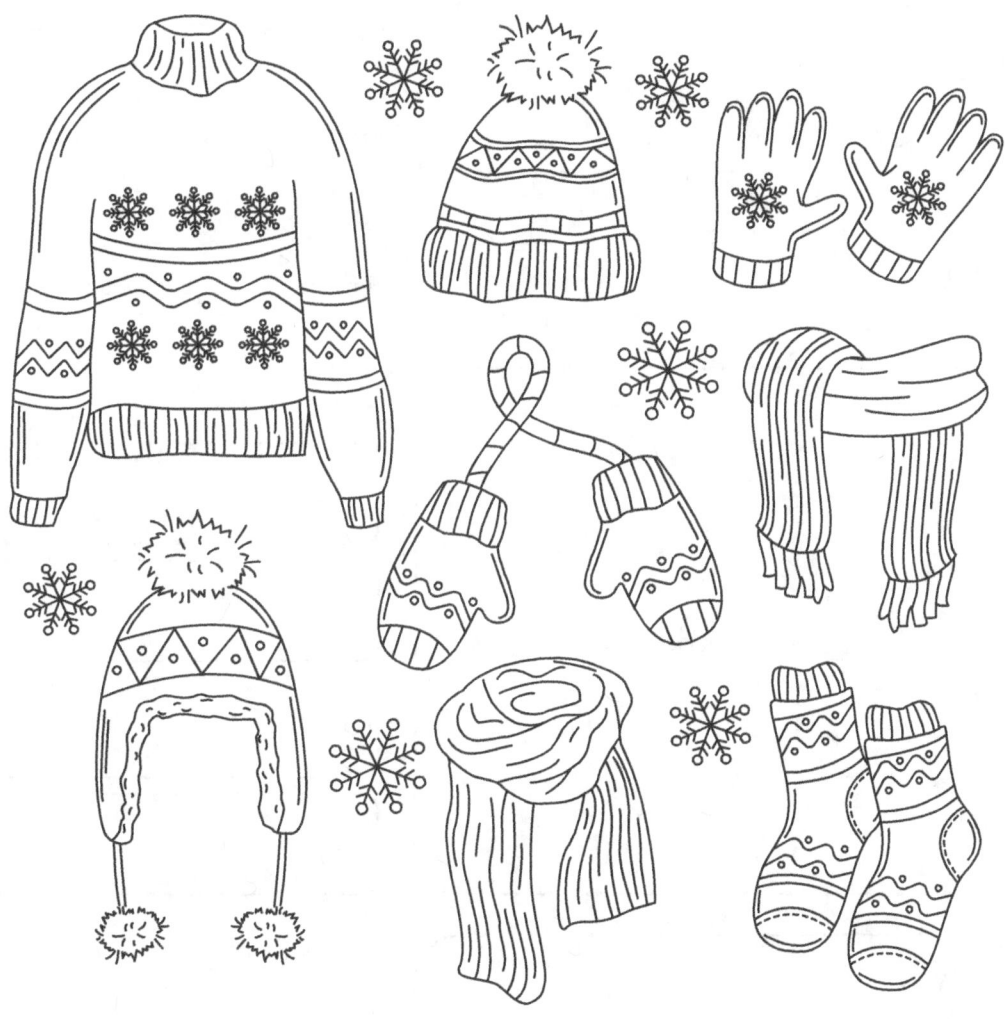

In knitting, you know how necessary it is to keep track of a single step of your project. That's where "My Knitting Project" comes in - a template that helps you plan and manage you knitting shots.

MY KNITTING TASK!

Task Name:

Pattern:

Patteren Source: Meter: Size:

Gauge: Hues: Starting Day and Date:

Needles: Required Amount: Finishing Day and Date:

My Idea!

The Colors!

1.

2.

3.

4.

My Notes!

My Ratings:

Pattern:

☆ ☆ ☆ ☆ ☆

Yarn:

☆ ☆ ☆ ☆ ☆

Overall Task:

☆ ☆ ☆ ☆ ☆

How fun was this task?

☆ ☆ ☆ ☆ ☆

1.2. Making a Personalized Picture Puzzle

This activity is incredibly excellent because it sparks creativity and remembrance.

Make a picture puzzle in 3 simple steps:

1. Make a copy of a favorite picture of your choice — like family, friend or a special place.
2. Cut the picture into puzzle-shaped segments. Ensure that the pieces are not too tiny and too many for handling.
3. Now shuffle all the parts and complete the puzzle.

Following is an example of a picture puzzle and how to cut it into pieces.

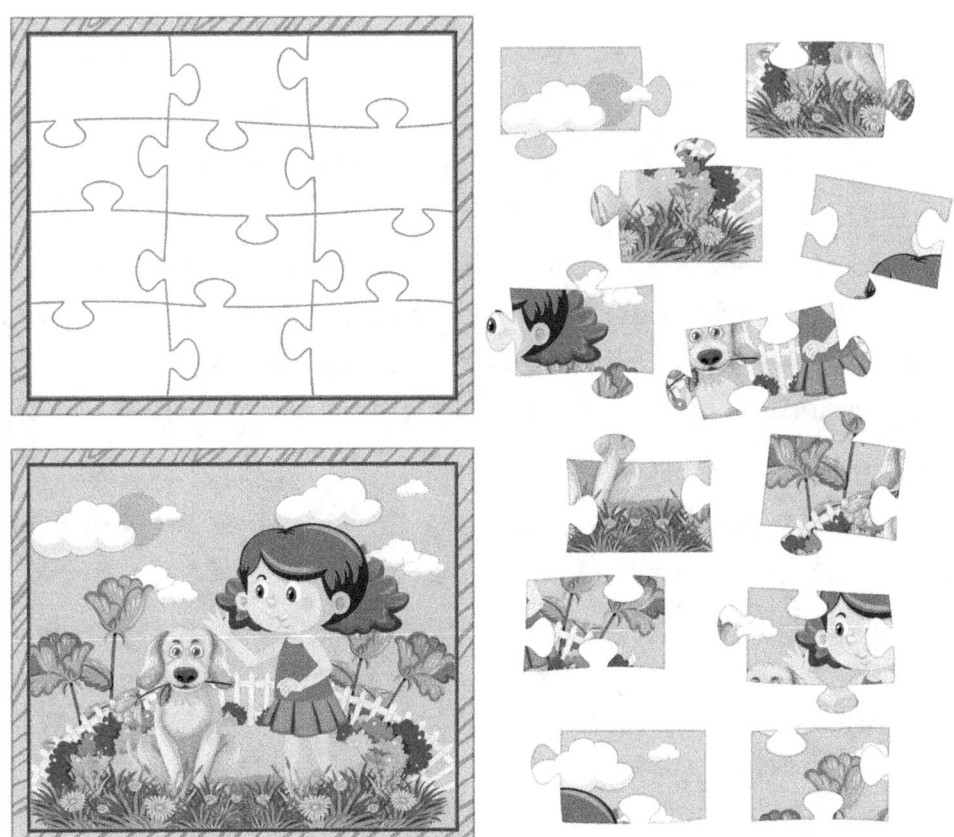

1.3. Drawing and Crafts

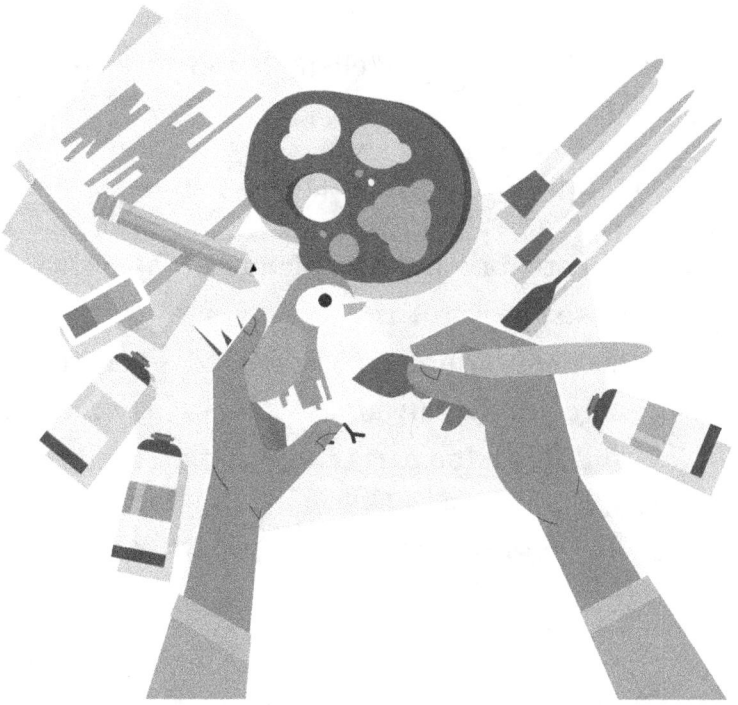

Being busy in arts and crafts is a delightful and practical mode of elevating and sustaining creativity via self-expression. Drawing, painting, ceramics and beading are easy and exciting projects you can relish. Art and crafts offer multiple benefits, like enhanced cognitive function, a sweetened mood, improved social dealings, and excellent self-expression. It can also enhance motor skills, relieve pain, forge fresh thought processes, and improve memory.

Art and crafts encourage you to create art and cultivate your senses, making it more comfortable to produce prompt neural connections that may have failed due to aging. It can reduce anxiety, depression, and tension levels, leading to positive shifts in your emotional health. Concentrating on drawing things and using pencils or paint can help you relax and focus on optimistic emotions, notably significant for stumbling with memory loss and hearing.

Art and crafts provide an alternative process of expression for you who may have challenges with articulated communication due to mental or physical corrosion. You can communicate yourself freely through multiple creative tasks. It can also help you deal with grief or serious medical issues and unlock a previously hidden passion.

Rehearsing arts can help those who are dealing with memory loss induced by dementia. Painting and drawings support discovering forgotten memories about loved ones and the past. It can also offer people living with memory loss a beat of clarity and the capacity to perform optimally. It may also assist with disorders linked with chronic pain, stimulating relaxation and reducing emotional distress.

You can meet like-minded people during outdoor art sessions to interact and connect regularly. These links can fight loneliness and improve your emotional health. Besides, when you practice skills like painting and drawing, you physically exercise your arms and hands, which can improve muscle coordination, increase blood flow, and develop better skills with time.

Exploring new movements and thoughts through art can help you think differently about life, reframing your perspectives and finding new joy. Practicing art and crafts is a powerful tool for you with dementia that can improve your well-being.

Before moving further, let's have an art break, and do this dot-to-dot drawing where you need to connect the dots and color the picture after completing it.

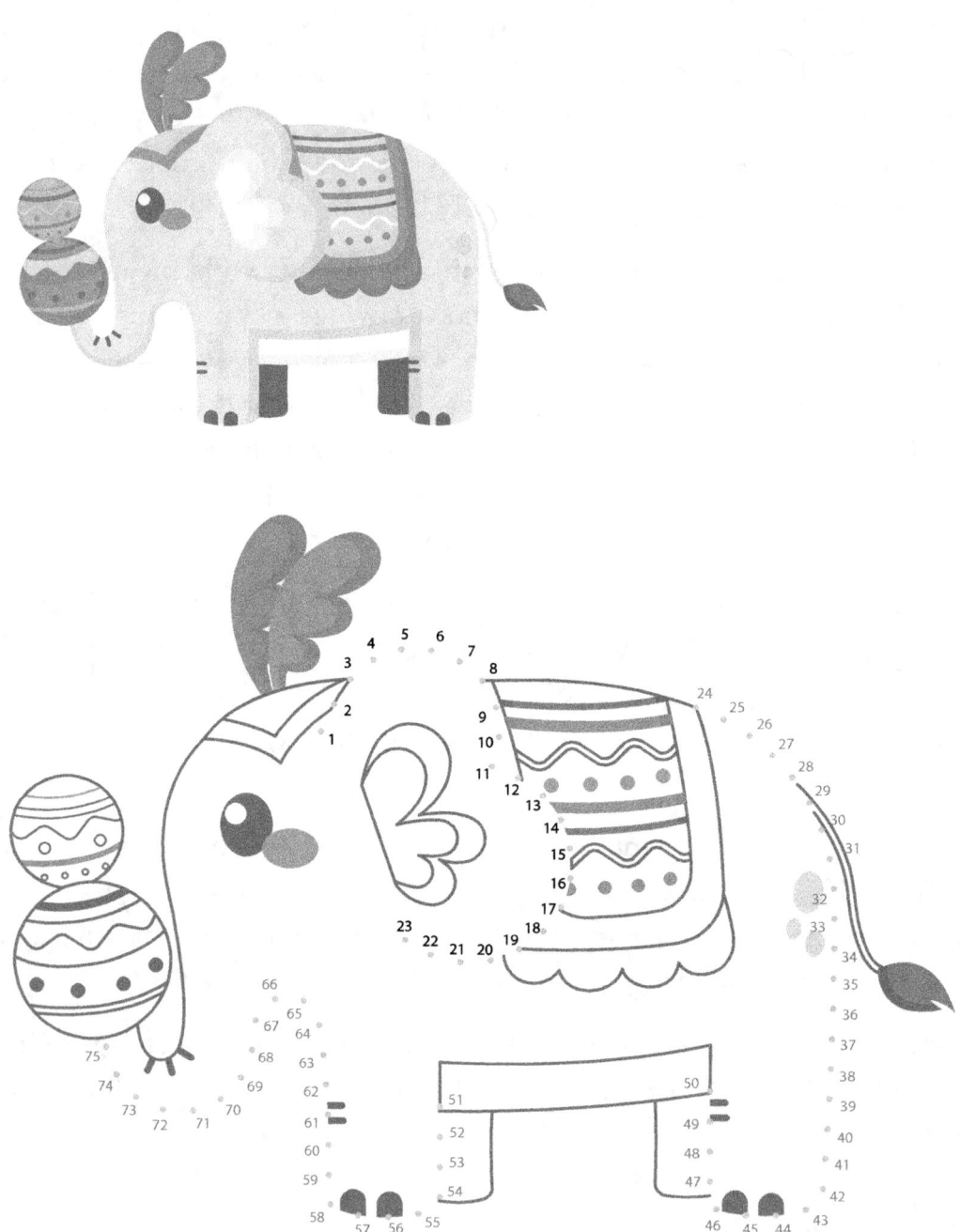

You can now engage in fun and creative peacock craft. This worksheet provides an easy, enjoyable, and perfect craft. You can assemble the parts and then color them according to your desire.

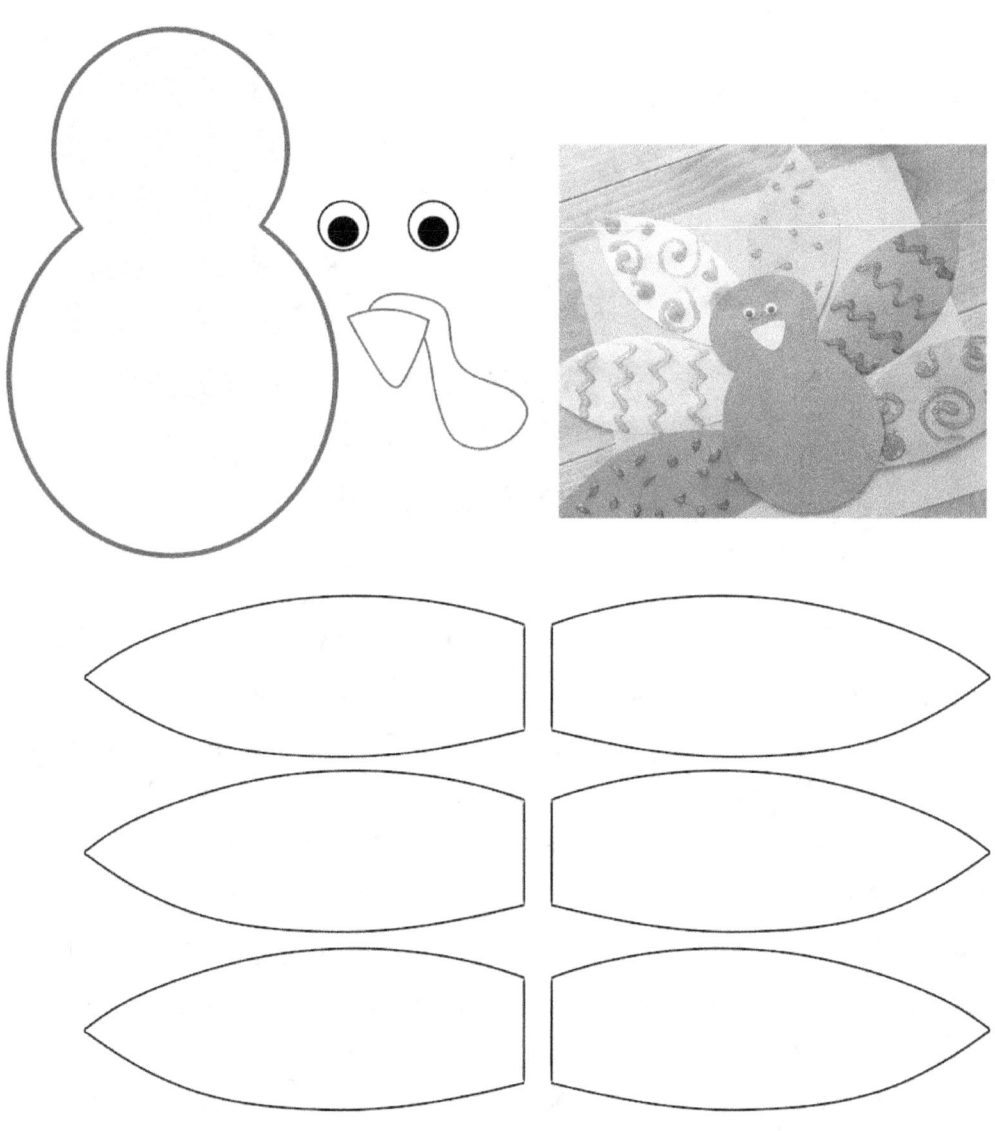

1.4. Mindfulness Break

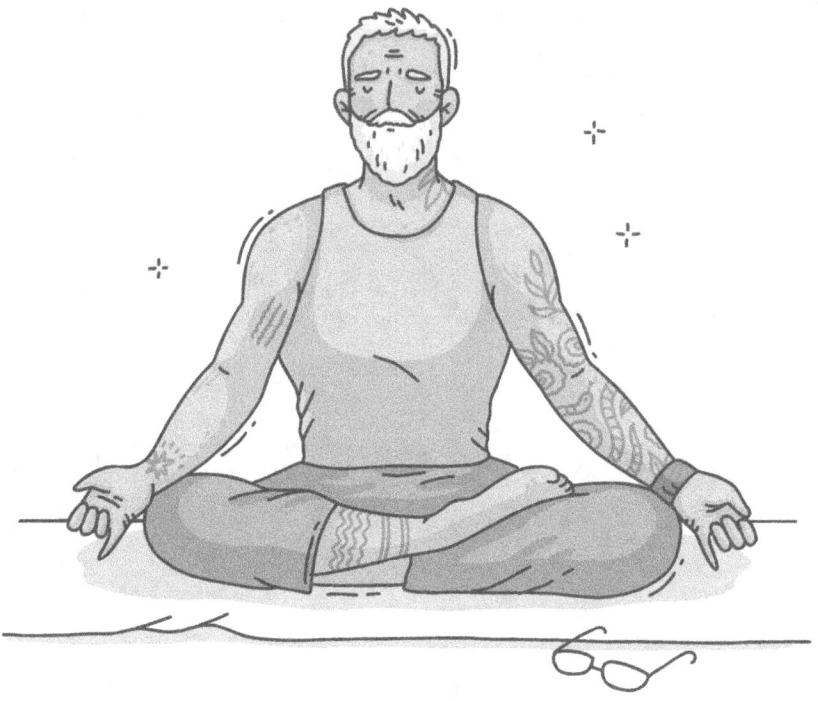

It's time to take a break and exercise mindfulness before proceeding to the next set of brain activities. Mindful breathing is a simple way to start this technique. Begin by locating a comfortable position, whether you prefer to sit, lie, or stand. Shut your eyes and concentrate on your inhales and exhales.

Attempt inhaling for 5 seconds, holding for 5 seconds, exhaling for 5 seconds, and then repeat. Focus on how your body reacts as you respire in and out. If your thoughts ramble, gently bring your focus back to your breath. You can continue this practice for as long as you are comfortable, but try for five minutes and then you can change the time with practice.

Bonus Brain Games

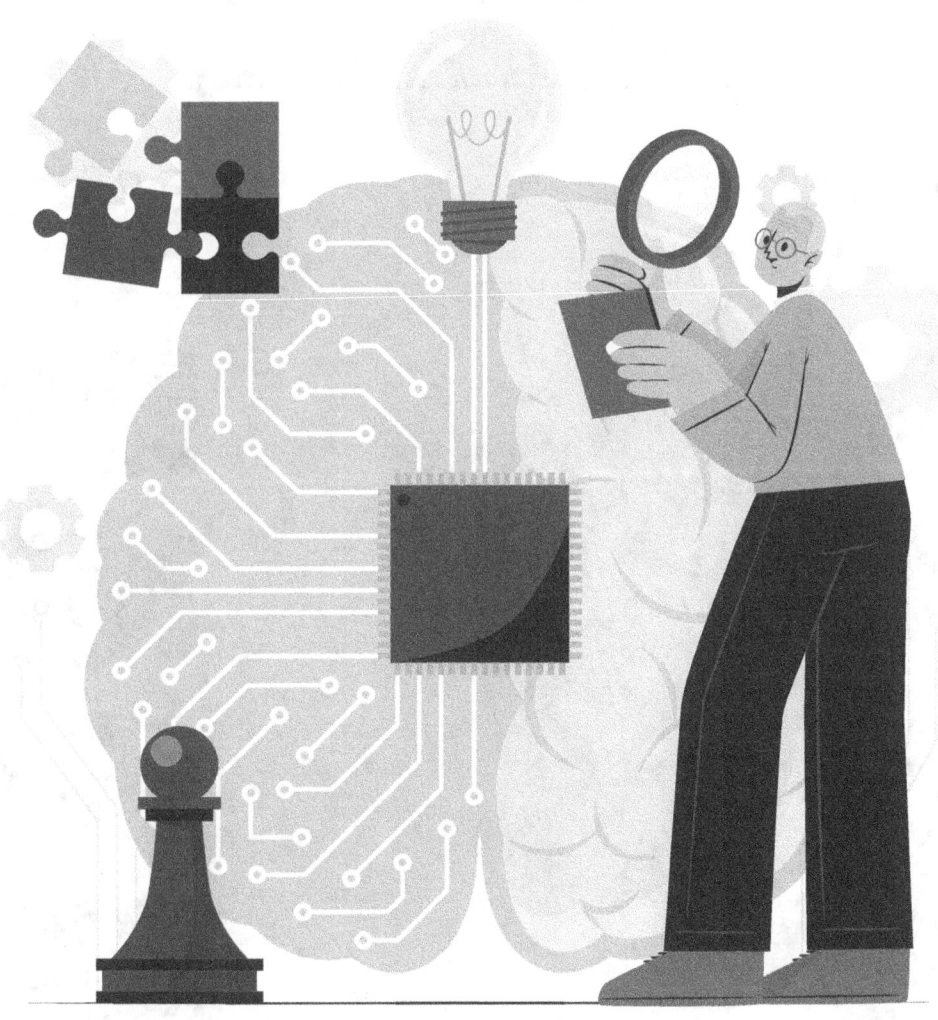

THE MITTEN MATCH

Match the mittens with respective patterns.

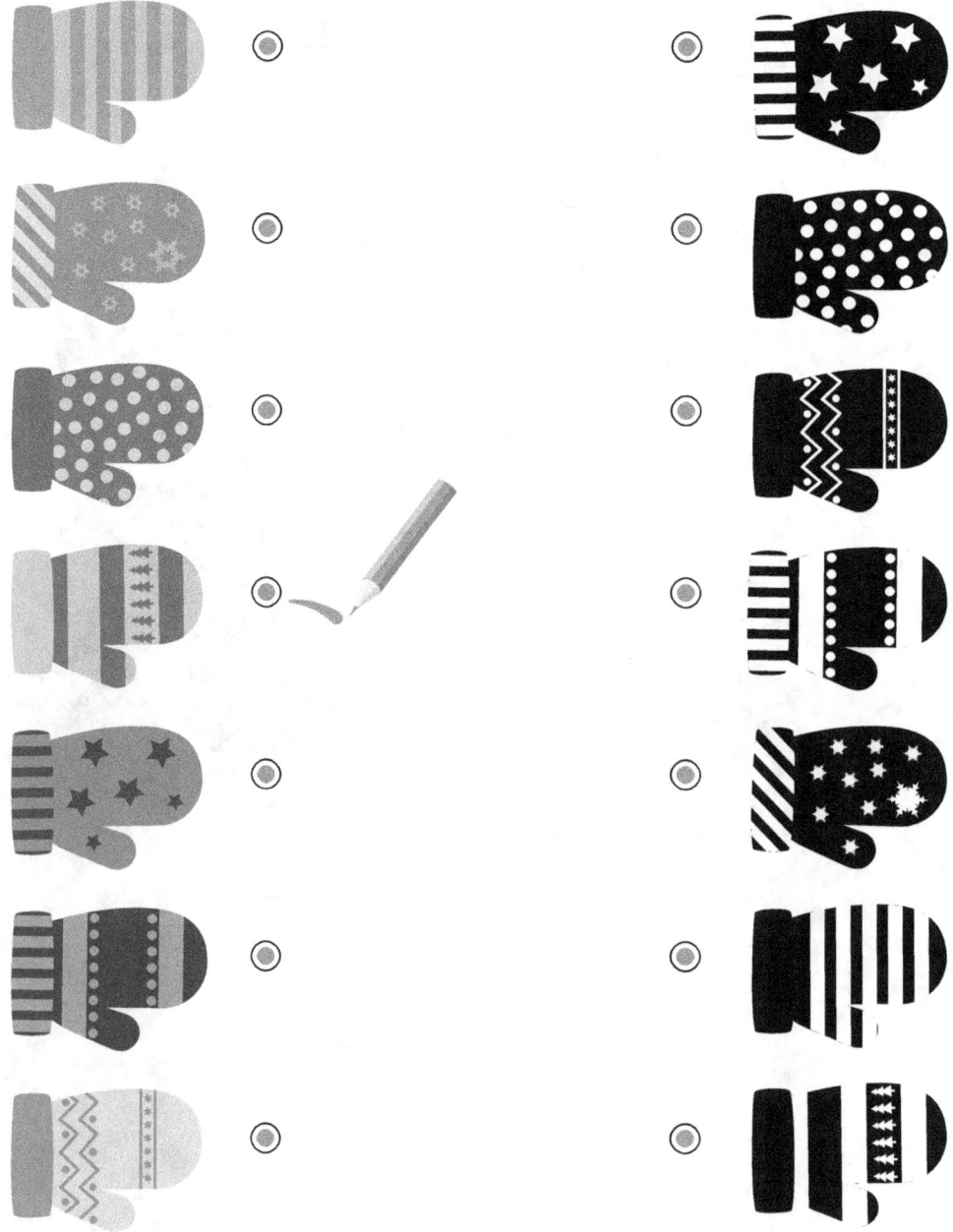

34

MATCH THE ASSOCIATED THINGS

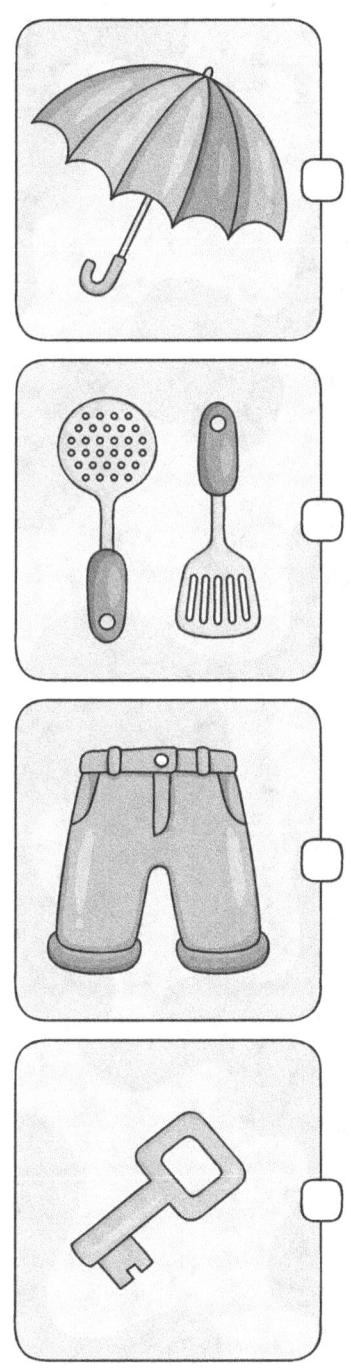
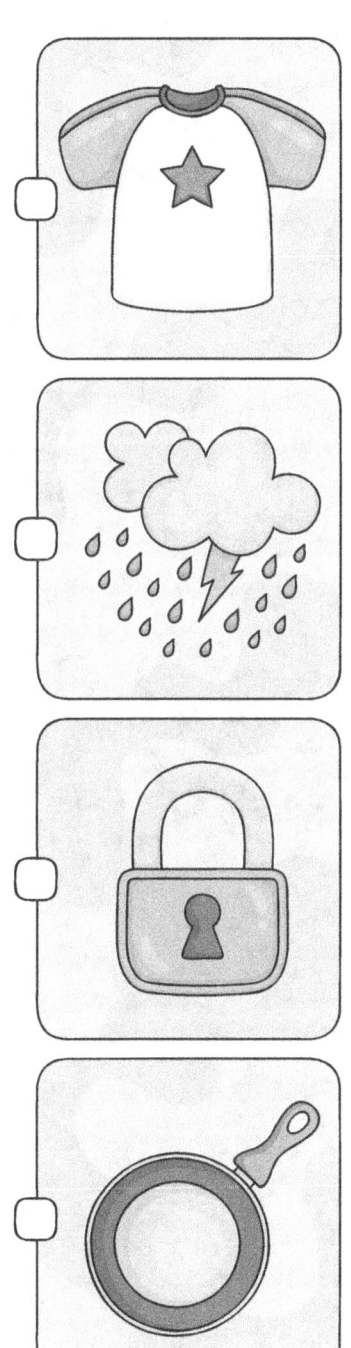

COLOR THE KNITTING KIT

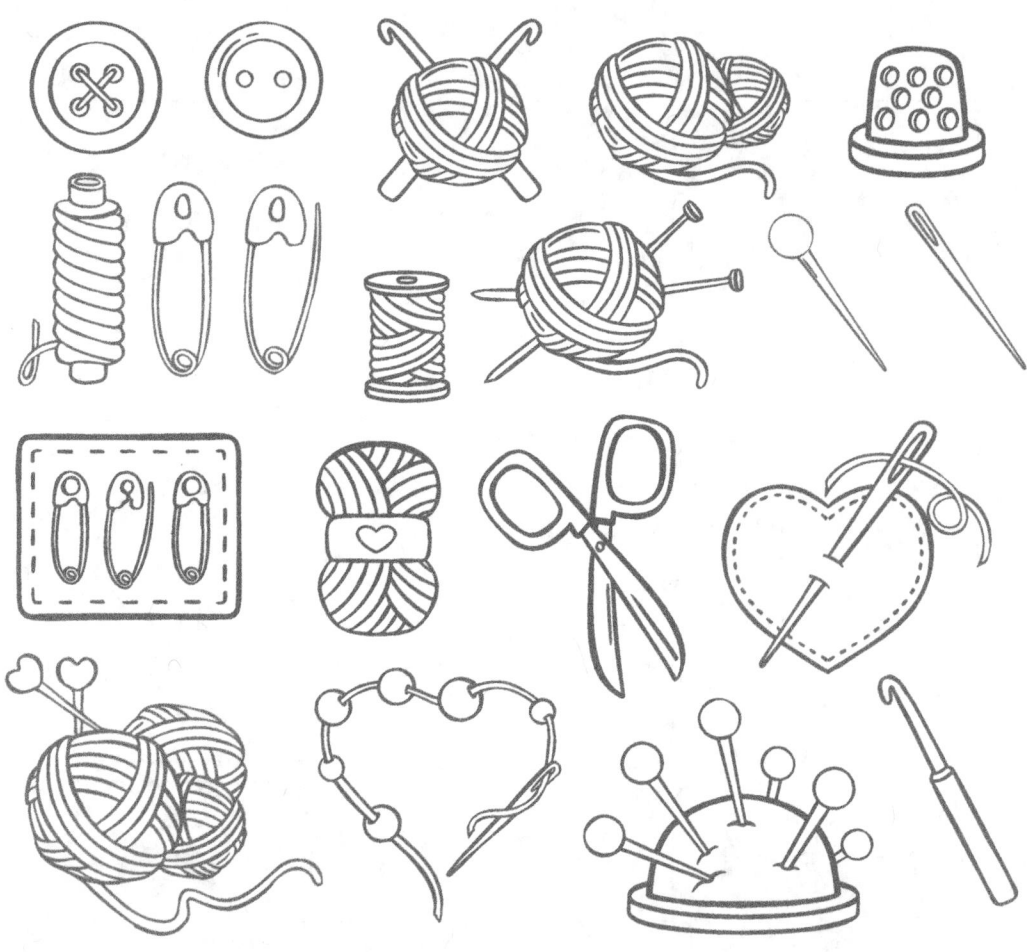

◆ **Counting: How Many**

COUNT THE KNIT STITCHES

Single stitch looks like this

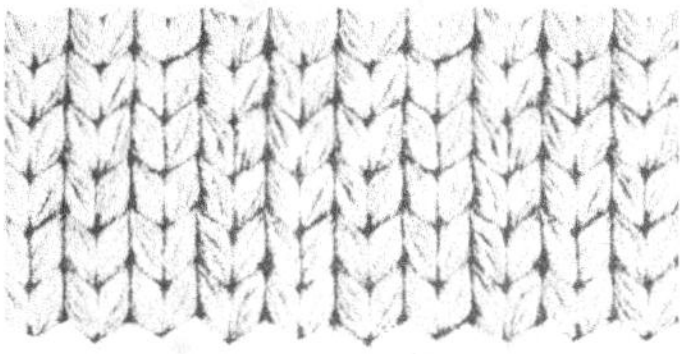

____________ Stitches

____________ Columns

____________ Rows

____________ Stitches

____________ Columns

____________ Rows

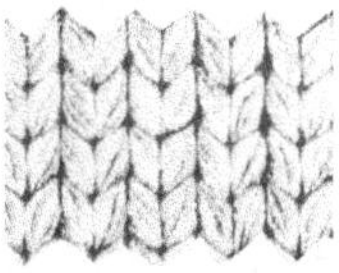

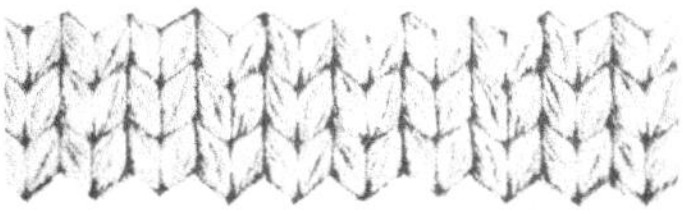

____________ Stitches

____________ Columns

____________ Rows

____________ Stitches

____________ Columns

____________ Rows

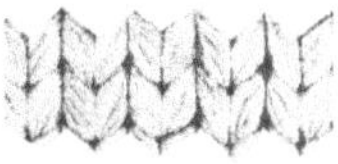

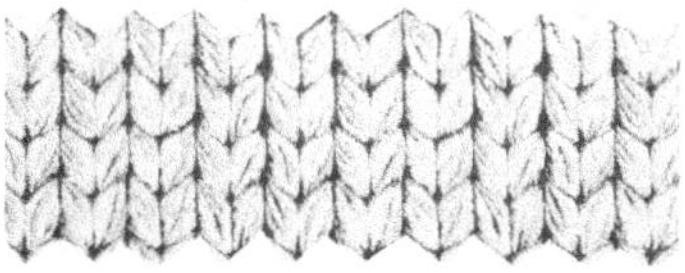

____________ Stitches

____________ Columns

____________ Rows

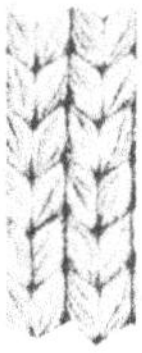

____________ Stitches

____________ Columns

____________ Rows

FRUIT COUNTING

Count the fruits.

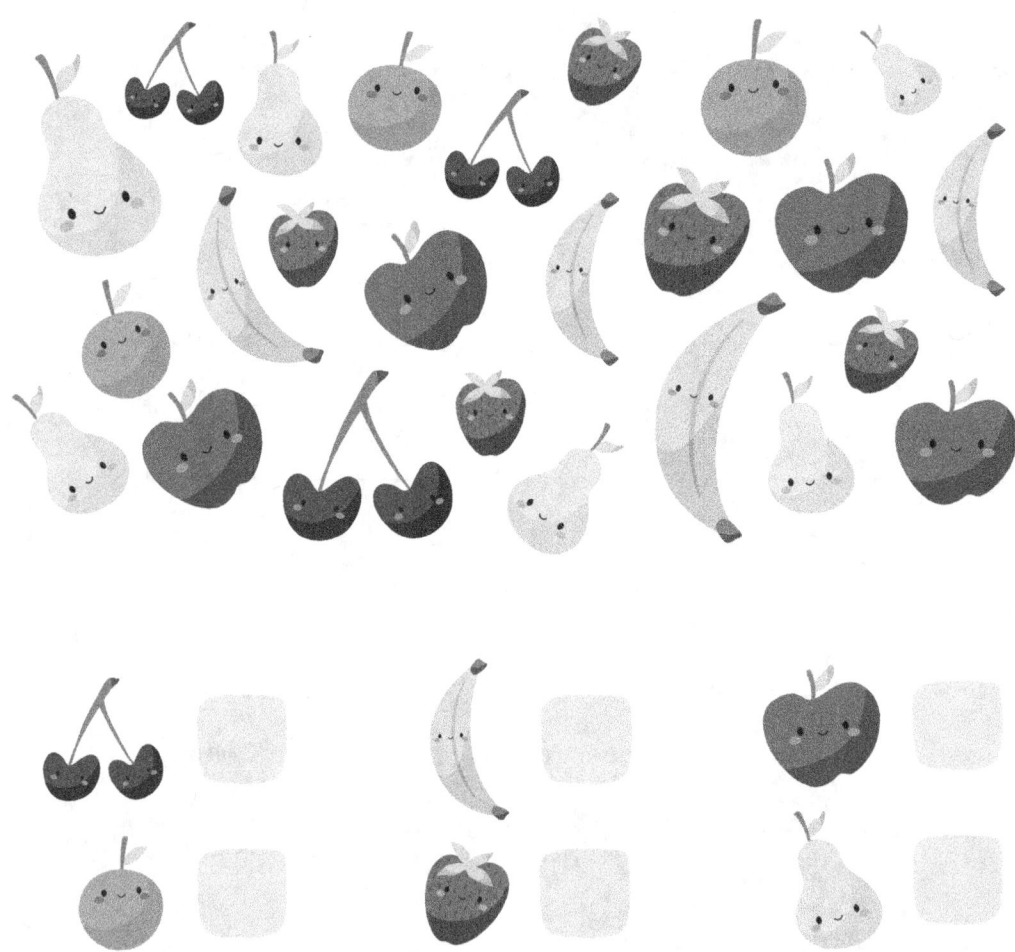

◆ Trivia

1. Which English king made Fair Isle pullovers trendy in the 1920s after resigning the throne to marry a divorcee?

_____

2. What is the finest stitch for a tight fit at the waist or wrist?

_____

3. What is the most typically used yarn weight for making socks?

_____

4. What is a pointed tool called that is used to make small holes?

_____

5. What is the art of folding paper to make object shapes called?

_____

6. What do you have if you make an artistic collection of materials and glue it to a surface?

_____

7. Which tool is commonly used when drawing a circle?

_____

8. Which artist is renowned for his fresco paintings?

_____

9. What are the three primary colors to consider when coloring?

_____

10. Name the secondary colors.

_____

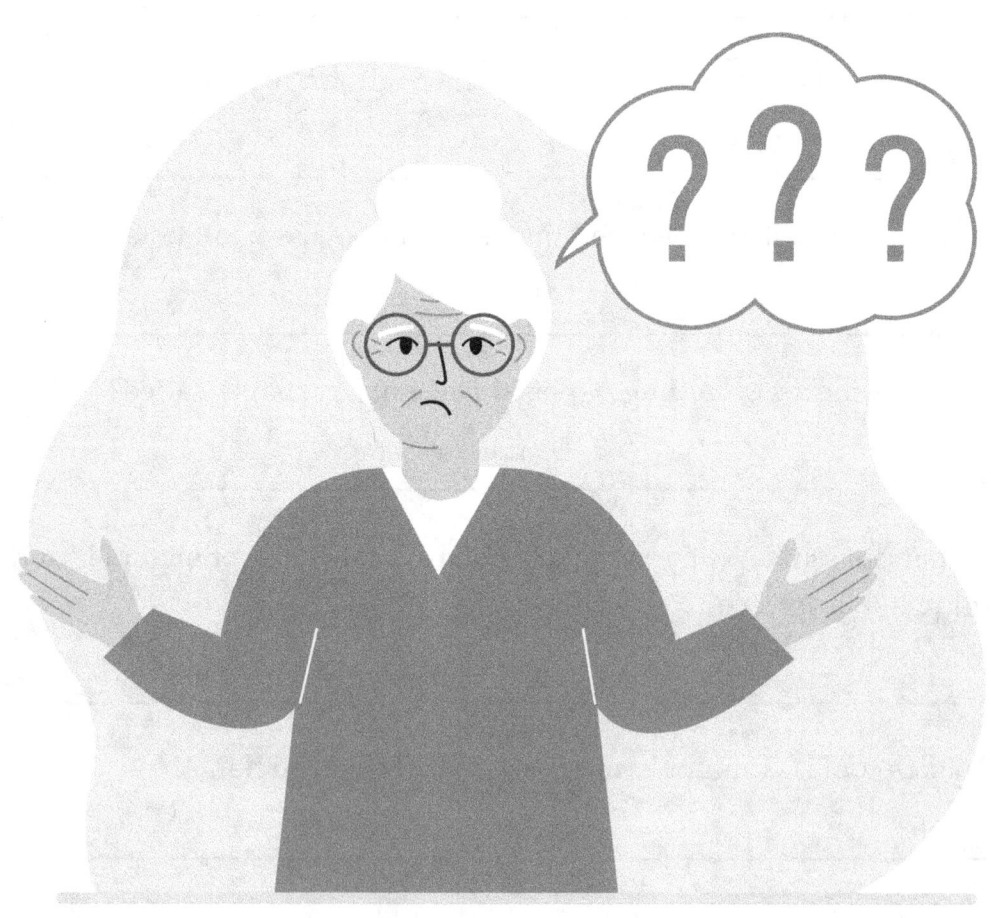

FINDING IDENTICAL DICES

Can you find two identical dice in the following worksheet?

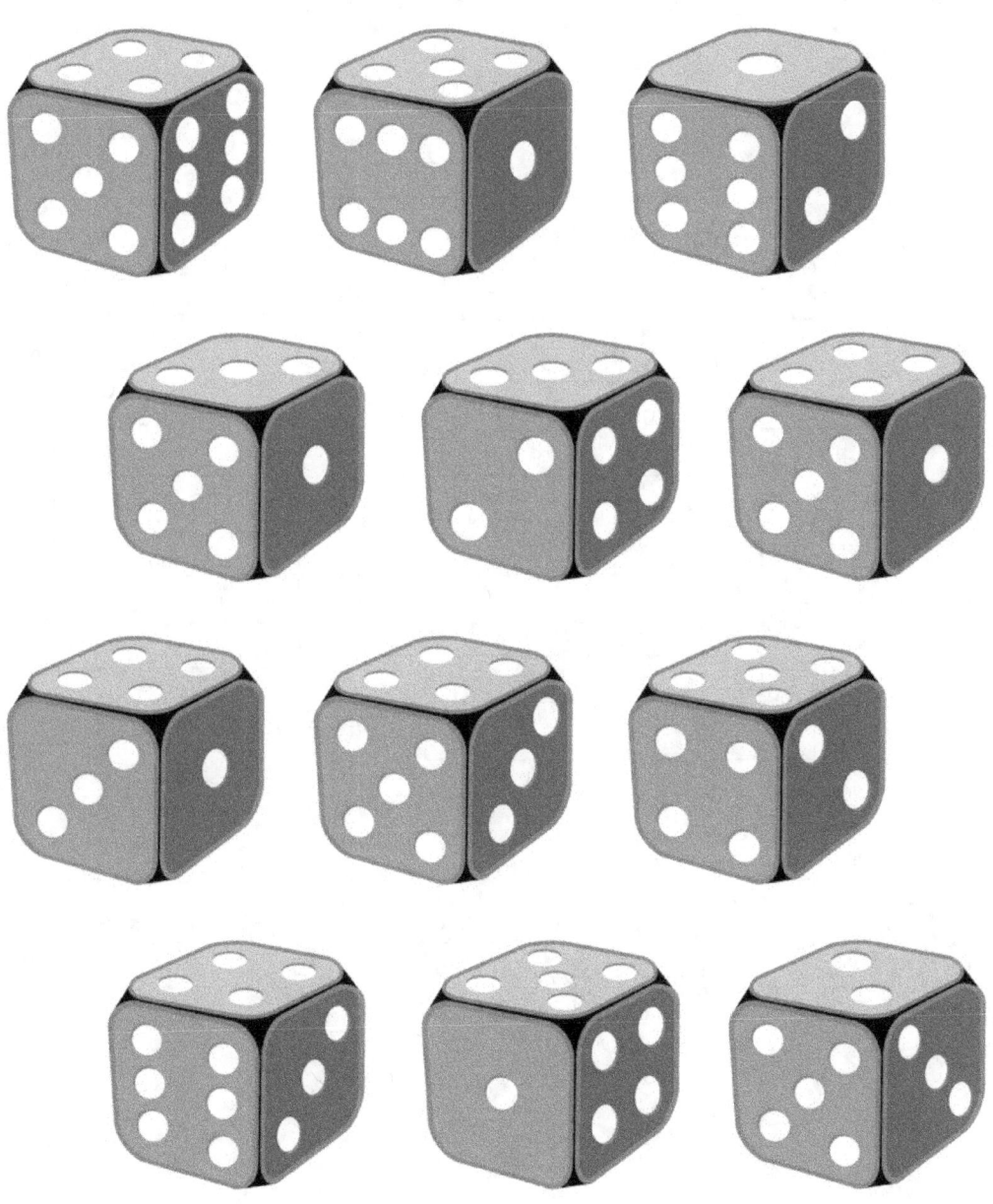

VISUAL PRACTICE

Follow the corresponding lines and color the fish.

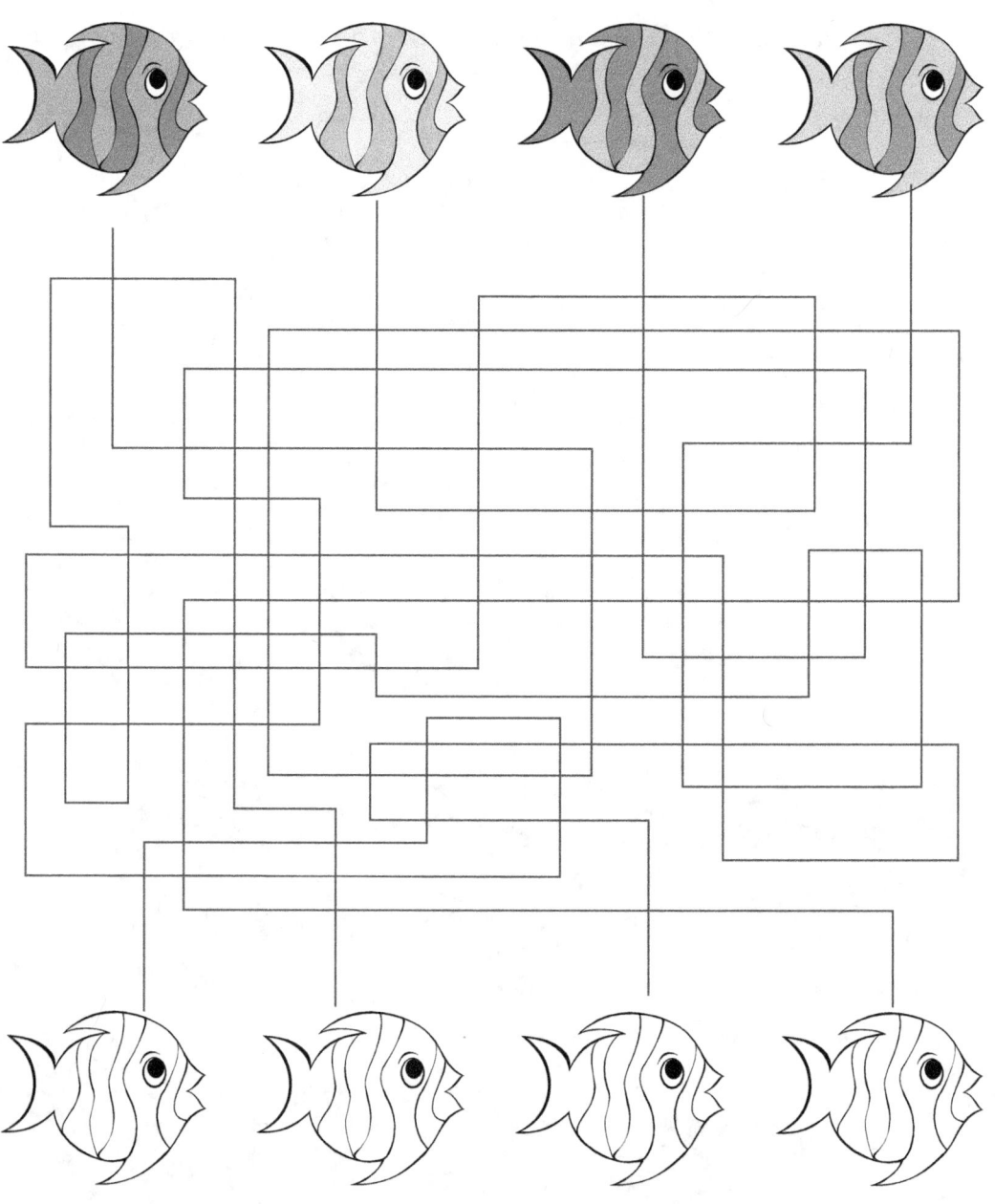

MISSING DOUBLES

Can you use two similar missing letters to finish each word?

A _ _ L E   M U _ _ I N

B R _ _ M   N _ _ N

C H E _ _ Y   O P O _ _ U M

D O _ _ A R   P I _ _ O W

E _ _ O R   Q U _ _ N

F O _ _ O W   S C I _ _ O R S

G I R A _ _ E   T E _ _ A C E

H I _ _ U P   U M B R E _ _ A

J E _ _ Y   V A _ _ E Y

K I _ _ E N   Y E _ _ O W

L I _ _ L E   Z I _ _ E R

BOGGLE

How many words can you create from the words given below?

E	B	S	L
T	H	A	W
G	Y	N	I
P	K	R	F

_____ _____ _____

_____ _____ _____

_____ _____ _____

_____ _____ _____

_____ _____ _____

TREE WORD SEARCH

```
W  A  T  F  O  L  I  A  G  E  S  H  O  T  E
P  C  B  R  A  N  C  H  S  O  N  E  P  V  L
T  A  H  A  B  Y  L  A  J  G  I  S  E  G  U
I  N  L  E  S  M  E  T  F  A  N  R  K  R  T
R  O  D  M  R  C  A  W  E  L  G  I  M  O  I
B  M  I  L  O  R  F  R  O  R  O  D  R  V  U
W  A  E  Y  T  X  Y  G  E  L  S  W  F  E  R
O  K  L  S  S  O  M  E  T  H  L  G  E  K  F
O  H  M  P  A  H  N  K  B  U  D  I  H  R  M
D  T  U  N  L  A  W  J  S  E  T  R  W  T  I
```

Search for tree-related words in all directions.

BRANCH	FOLIAGE	PALM
BUD	FRUIT	RINGS
CHERRY	GROVE	WALNUT
ELM	LEAF	WILLOW
EVERGREEN	LIMB	WOOD
FLOWER	MOSS	

1960s FAVORITE TV SHOWS

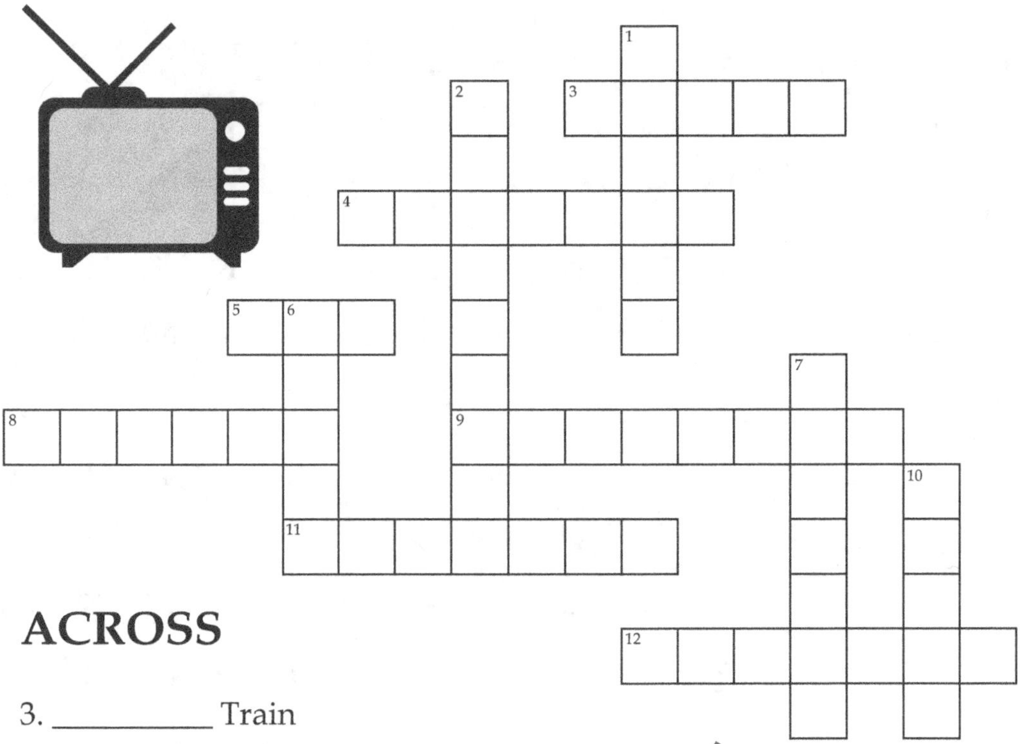

ACROSS

3. _____ Train

4. Wild _____

5. The _____ Patrol

8. Family _____

9. Love, _____ Style

11. Dark _____

12. Hollywood _____

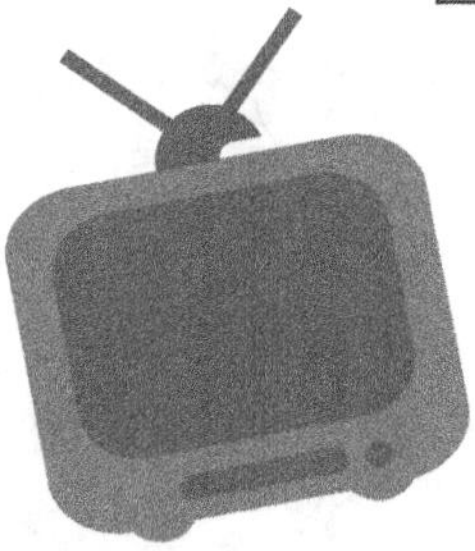

DOWN

1. _____ Adventures of
   Mr. Magoo

2. American _____

6. Green _____

7. My Favorite _____

10. The _____ Limits

SUDOKU PUZZLE

Fill in the blank spaces with numbers from 1 to 7.

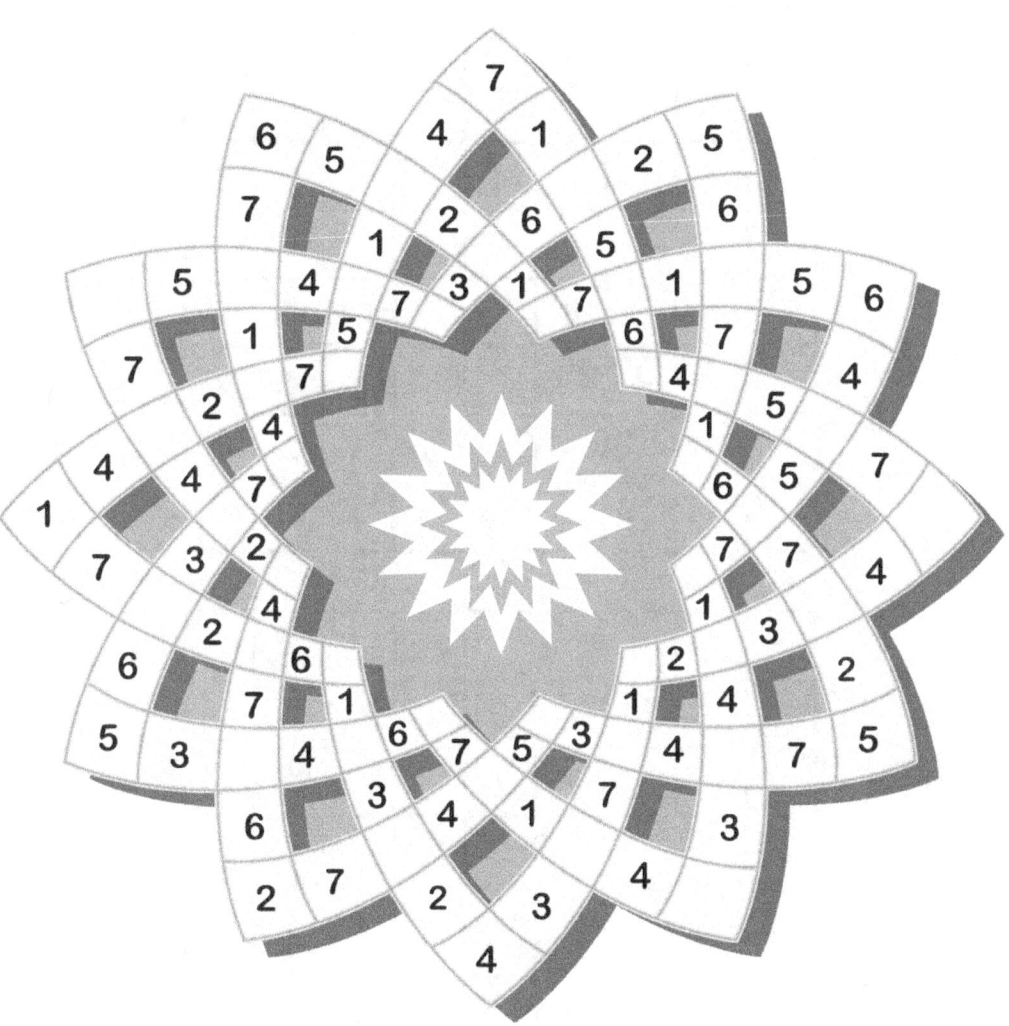

Place the numbers 1 - 9 exactly once in each row, column, and 3x3 region.

Puzzle 1

8						2	6	
			3	4	7			
	3	5		7				
	9							5
	1			6		9		
		8				2	7	
	4	3				9		
	1				9			6
						4		

Puzzle 2

	5						9	4
				5				
			7	1				
5						2		
							4	
		6		9	4	3		7
				2			8	
8	9				6	1	3	
2			9				6	

NUMBER PATTERNS WORKSHEET

Complete the patterns by writing the next number.

2	4	6	8				

1	3	5	7				

10	15	20	25				

12	16	20	24				

21	26	31					

13	18	23					

33	36						

SHAPE PATTERNS WORKSHEET

Guess which shape comes next and then color it.

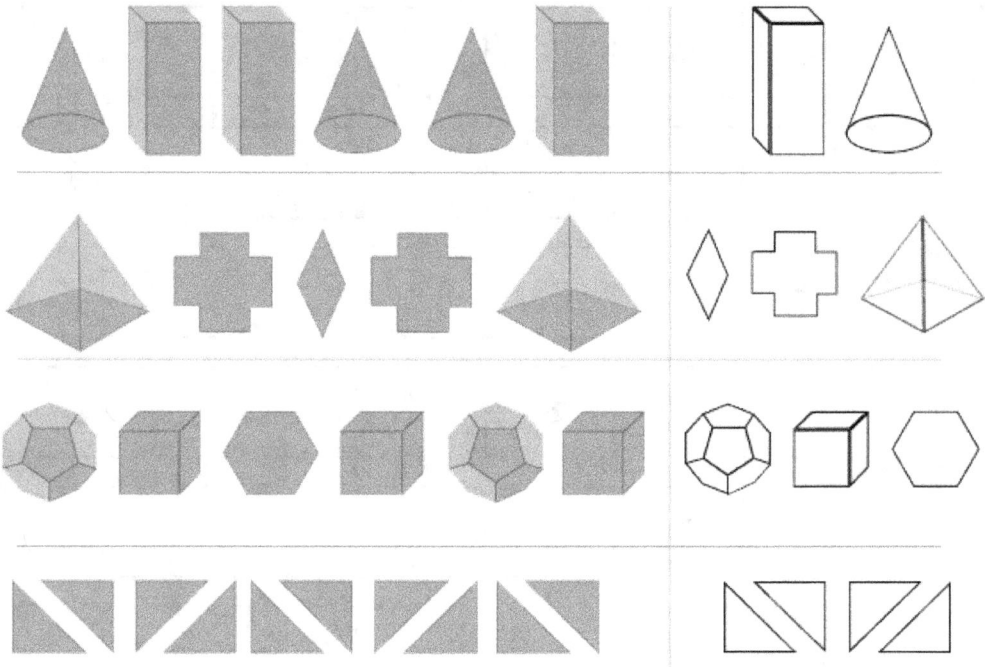

WORD ASSOCIATION GAME

What comes to your mind when you hear...?

Read and complete this word association game.

School   _____   _____

Ocean   _____   _____

Hospital   _____   _____

Music   _____   _____

Rocking chair   _____   _____

U.S.A.   _____   _____

Apple   _____   _____

Life   _____   _____

Bicycles   _____   _____

Government   _____   _____

Forest   _____   _____

Mobile   _____   _____

Park   _____   _____

Grandchildren   _____   _____

Science   _____   _____

Hiking   _____   _____

Fishing   _____   _____

Gossip   _____   _____

WORD ASSOCIATION FAMILY TIME

1- AFTER READING THE WORDS ON THE LEFT COLUMN, JOT DOWN THE FIRST THING THAT COMES TO YOUR MIND.
2- ASK A FAMILY MEMBER WHAT COMES TO THEIR MIND BY USING THE QUESTION "WHAT COMES TO YOUR MIND WHEN YOU THINK OF....".

WORD	I Think Of	My Family Member Thinks Of
Spouse		
Red		
Shopping		
Sunday		
Ice Cream		
Holiday		
Beach		
Long Drive		
Money		
Yoga		

PART - II
2. Sensory Activities for Seniors Coping with Dementia

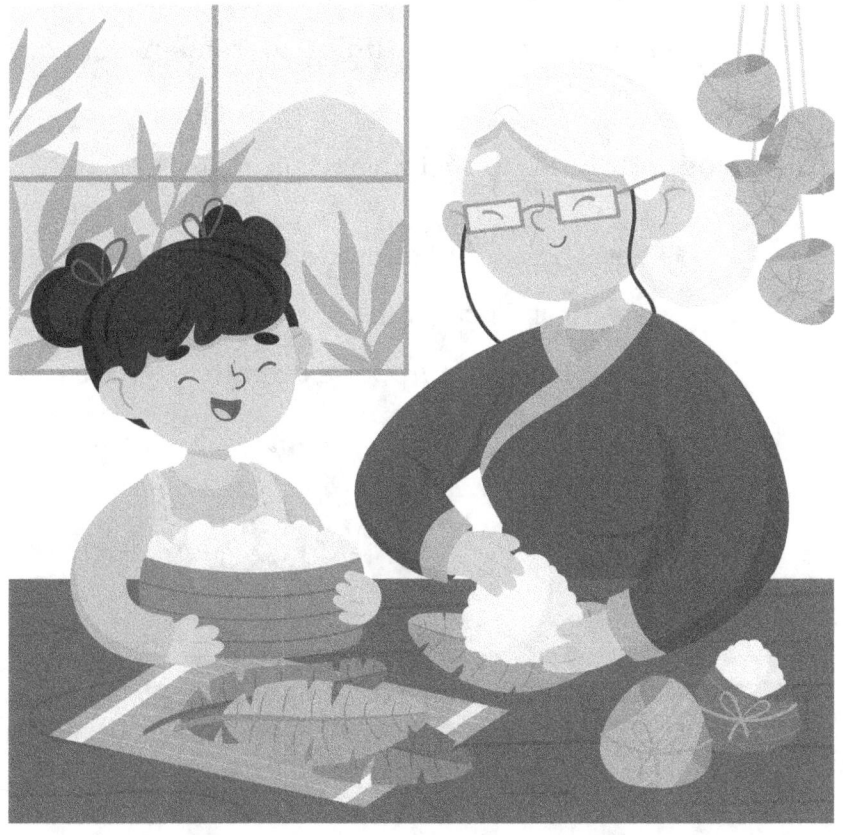

You may have noticed a slight decrease in logical reasoning and speech over time, even when you have your physical senses.

Sensory stimulation comprises any activity or venture that stimulates 1 of the 5 senses:

1. Sight
2. Smell
3. Touch
4. Taste
5. Sound

Sensory activities are designed to help you because they:

✓ Come up with cognitive and touchable stimulation via creativity.

✓ Allow personal responsibility by keeping a sense of self.

✓ Provide you with the opportunity to remain connected and engaged.

✓ Furnish opportunities to sustain and promote

- The variety of motion
- Resilience; and
- Mastery of upper-extremity exercises

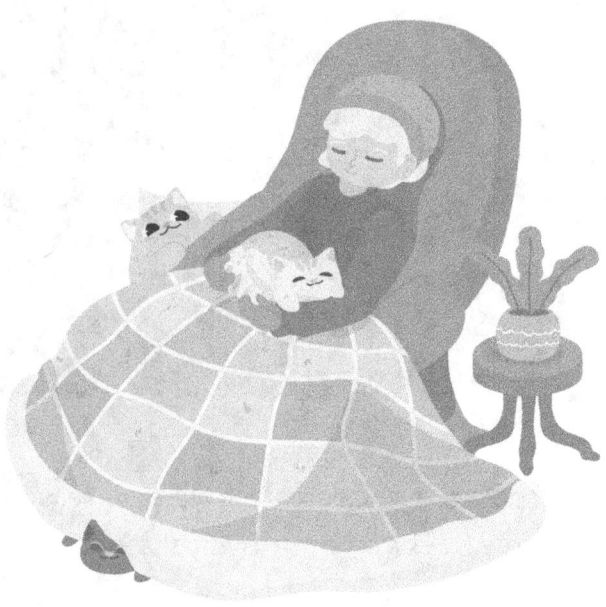

2.1. Culinary Activities

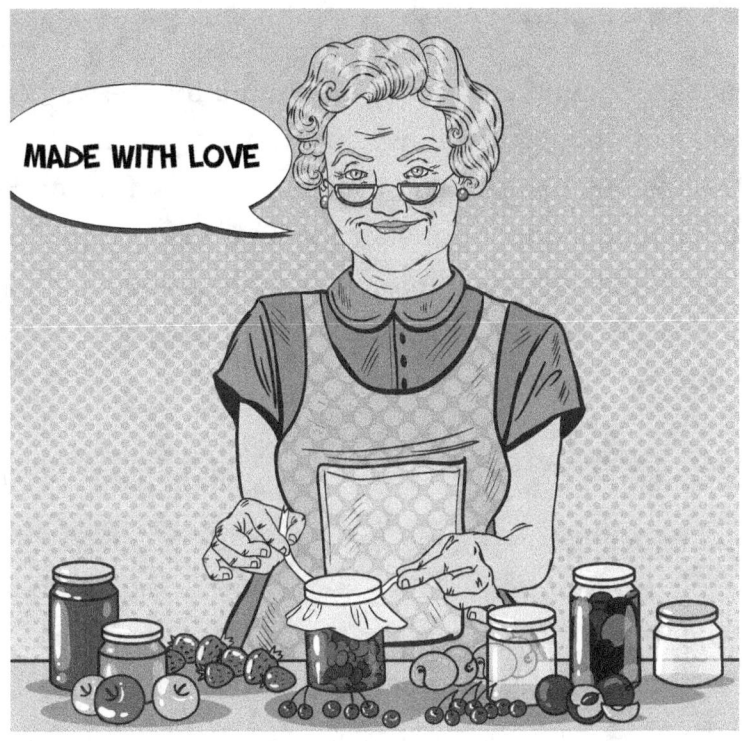

If you are a food lover, culinary activities can be a superb way to satisfy your interest and activate your senses. Above all, it's satisfy, and no fancy things are required.

You may relish making a classic meal if you are a home chef.

An activity that all can appreciate is baking. The kneading and rolling of dough can promote the tangible senses.

You can try:

- Cake
- Biscuits
- Pies

The aroma of these freshly baked things will provoke the appetite, when dispersed around the house, welcoming your family to your tea table.

1. Prepare a fruit salad

Preparing salads is an excellent way of stimulating the senses and it has several stages: selecting the fruit, washing it, and peeling it. While doing these small activities, you should smell and feel the fruit and talk about its smell, flavor and shape. Allow family members to introduce unusual exotic fruits and discuss where the fruits globally come from. Also, dig up the memories and share what fruit you ate when you were younger. Encourage others to taste your salad.

2. Make sandwiches

Sandwiches are healthy and good food item to try. They also consist of multiple steps: first, buttering the bread, spreading sandwich fillings that can be anything like your favorite veggies, boiled chicken, egg, or mayonnaise, and finally, setting the sandwiches on a plate.

3. Ice and decorate cupcakes, biscuits or Easter eggs

Pre-made icing and handy squeeze tubes in various colors are available in the market.

Connect your activity to a theme or an occasion such as Easter, Halloween, bonfire night, Christmas, or birthday of your loved ones. Decorate cupcakes and biscuits with these colorful, easy-to-use icing. Adding sprinkles, choco chips or fresh fruits can add variety to them.

4. Help in cooking

You can also help a person who is cooking in the kitchen by participating in simple tasks such as:

- Stir dessert, bake potatoes or make stew in a pan.
- Add extras such as marmalade to rice pudding.
- Offer gravy onto other meal.
- Finger slice the bread or toast to dip into a stew or to be offered with an egg.

Trust me; your family will be happy to look on. Still, you can have an opportunity to smell and look at the meal as it is being prepared.

5. Involvement in Meal Serving

You can also be a part of different chores associated with arranging a meal – making the table, for instance – which can help you memorize skills and increase your confidence. Laying the table may apply to putting out cutlery like knives and forks, placing mats, and folding napkins. After enjoying the meal, other chores follow:

- Removing the plates and crockery
- Cleaning the table
- Dish washing
- Drying plates and pots
- Organizing the utensils

A person with dementia may enjoy participating in any one or all of these tasks. You can make your drinks or help others to make theirs. Some of you may enjoy one part, like adding the sugar into a cup or the teabags into a teapot.

My dear seniors, it's time to have some heart-to-heart conversation about food.

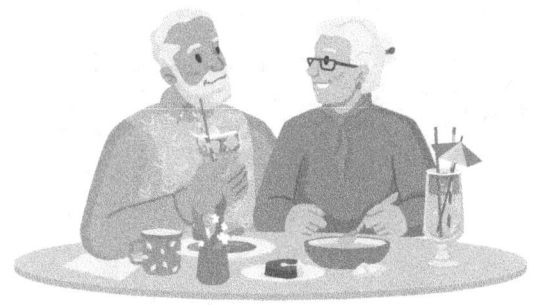

CONVERSATION ABOUT FOOD

We know food is an excellent topic for conversation. Let's have some conversation and tell us a few things.

1. Please tell us how you prefer tea or coffee in a cup or mug.

_____

2. Where do you go for groceries?

_____

3. What day do you prefer to go to the market?

_____

4. What mode of transportation do you choose?

_____

5. What is your signature dish? Why?

_____

6. What were your favorite candies as a child?

_____

To make your life easier, here are a few easy-to-cook recipes you can make without assistance.

Sangria

The Spanish Delight

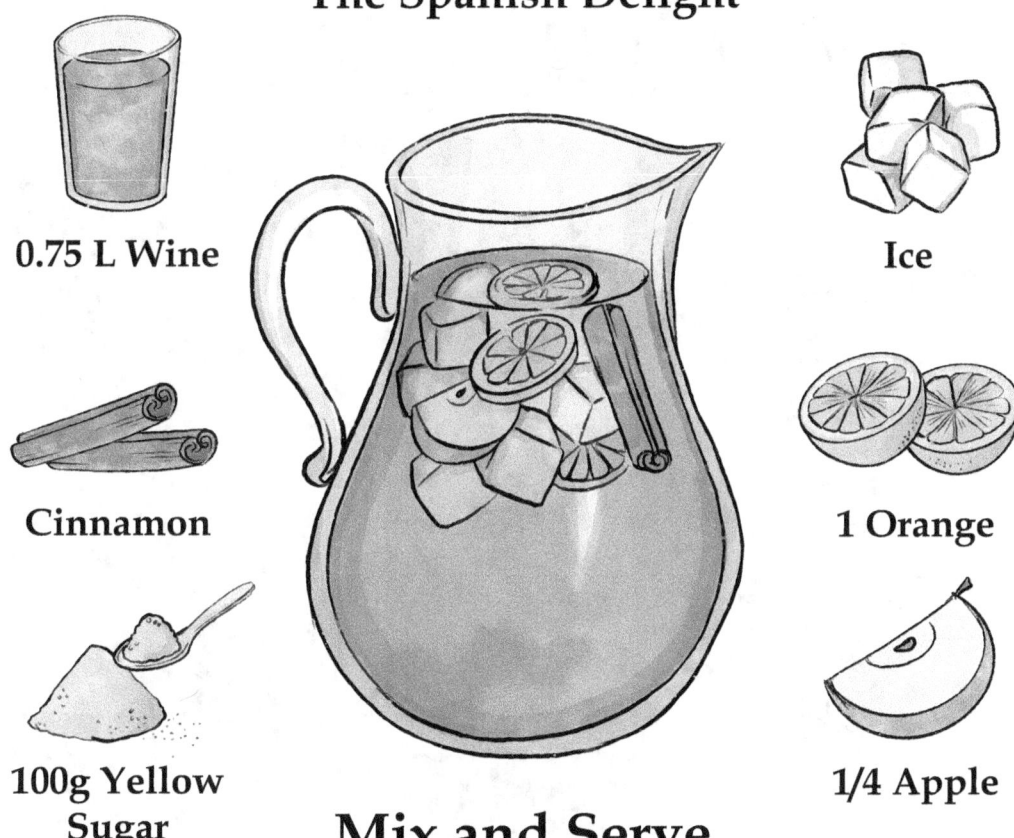

0.75 L Wine

Cinnamon

100g Yellow
Sugar

Ice

1 Orange

1/4 Apple

Mix and Serve

RED BERRY SMOOTHIE

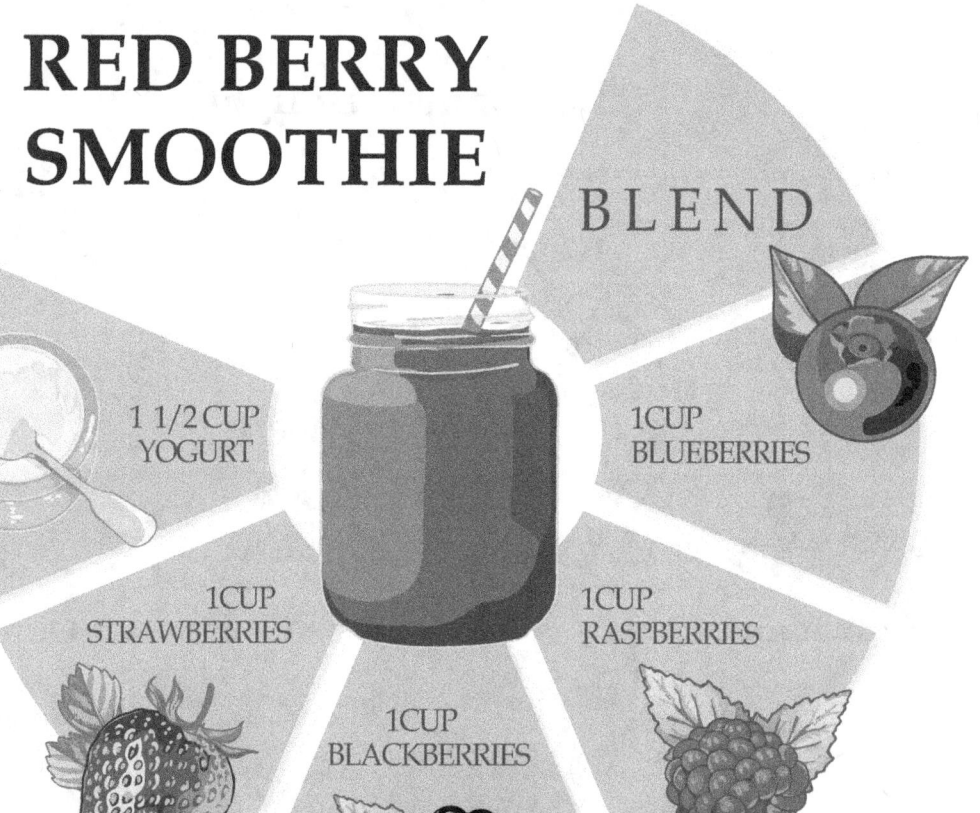

BLEND

1 1/2 CUP YOGURT

1CUP BLUEBERRIES

1CUP STRAWBERRIES

1CUP RASPBERRIES

1CUP BLACKBERRIES

HOMEMADE BREAD

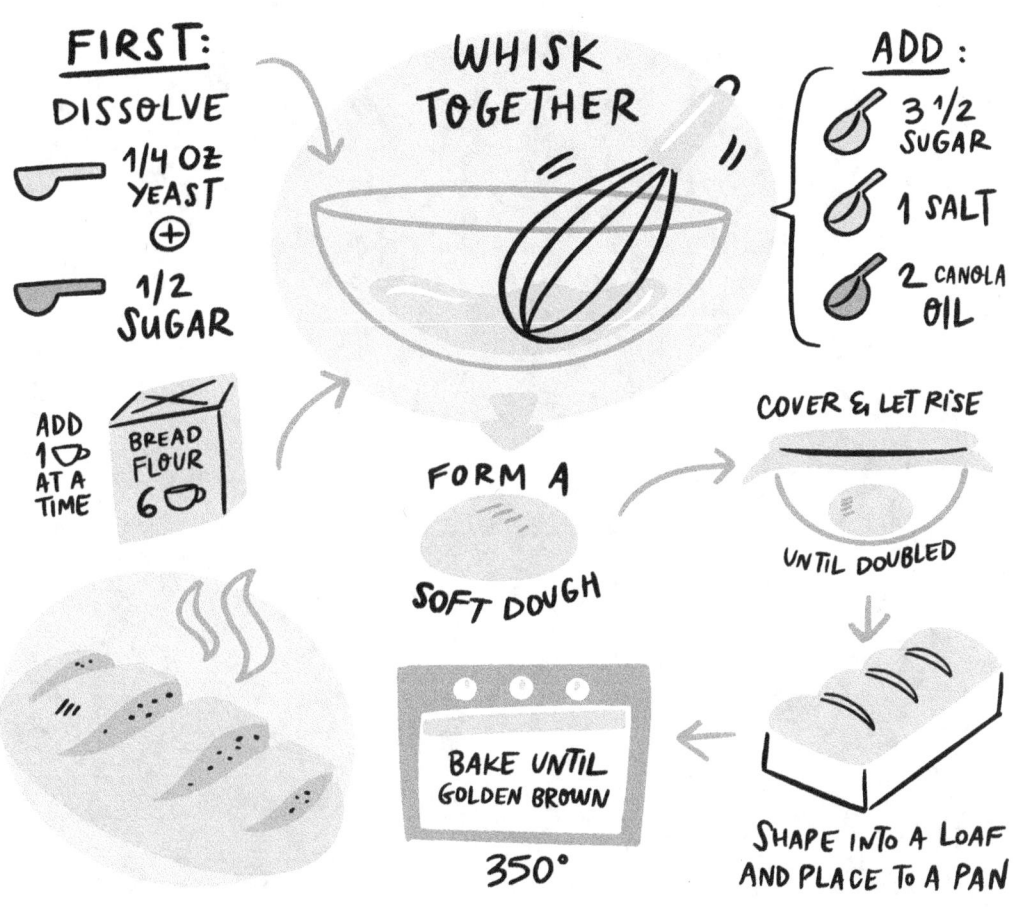

FIRST:
DISSOLVE
1/4 OZ YEAST
⊕
1/2 SUGAR

ADD 1 AT A TIME
BREAD FLOUR 6

WHISK TOGETHER

ADD:
3 1/2 SUGAR
1 SALT
2 CANOLA OIL

FORM A
SOFT DOUGH

COVER & LET RISE
UNTIL DOUBLED

SHAPE INTO A LOAF AND PLACE TO A PAN

BAKE UNTIL GOLDEN BROWN
350°

Now it's your turn to share your best recipe with us; try to recall all the ingredients and jot them down in the following sheet.

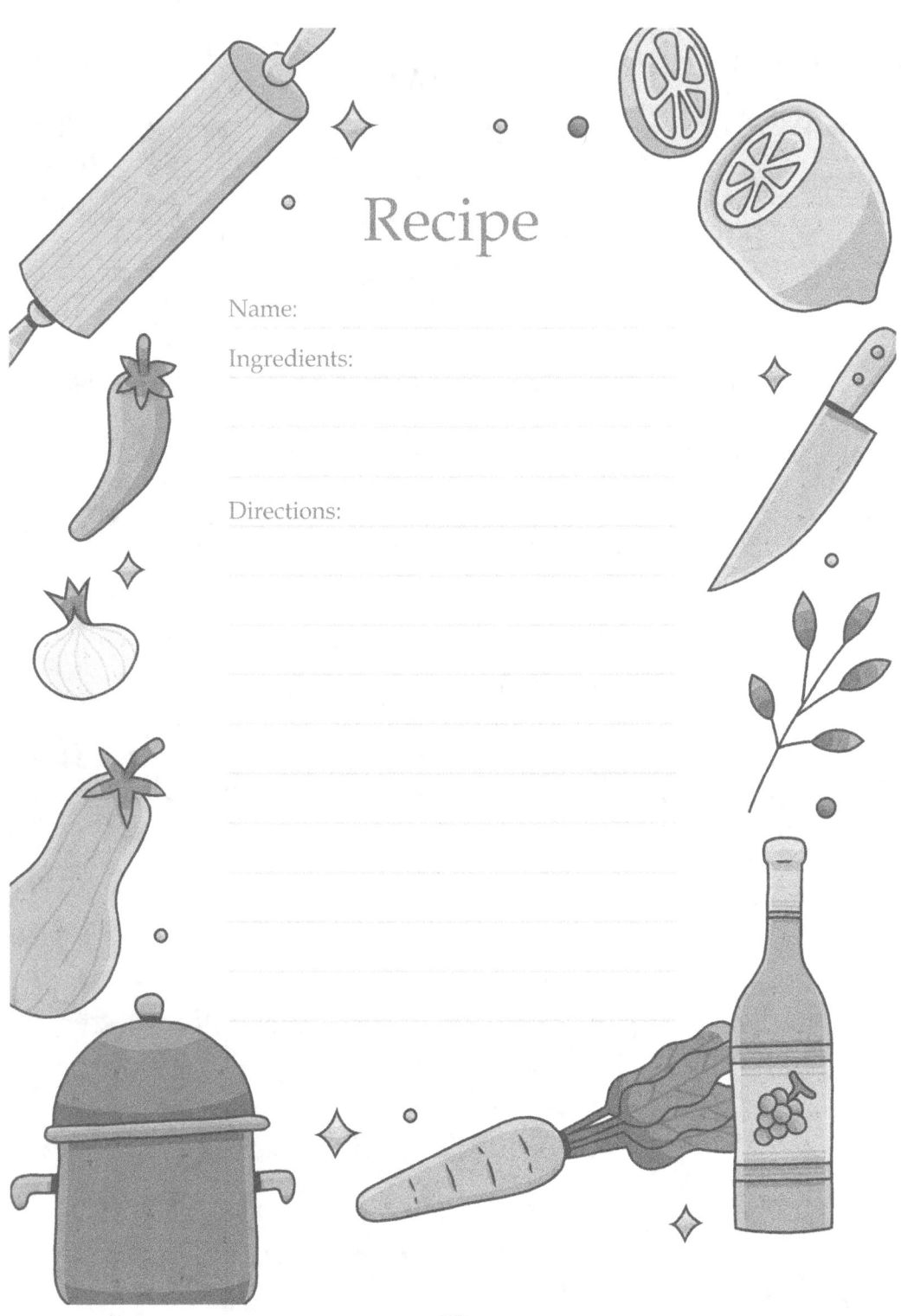

Recipe

Name:

Ingredients:

Directions:

2.2. Folding Laundry

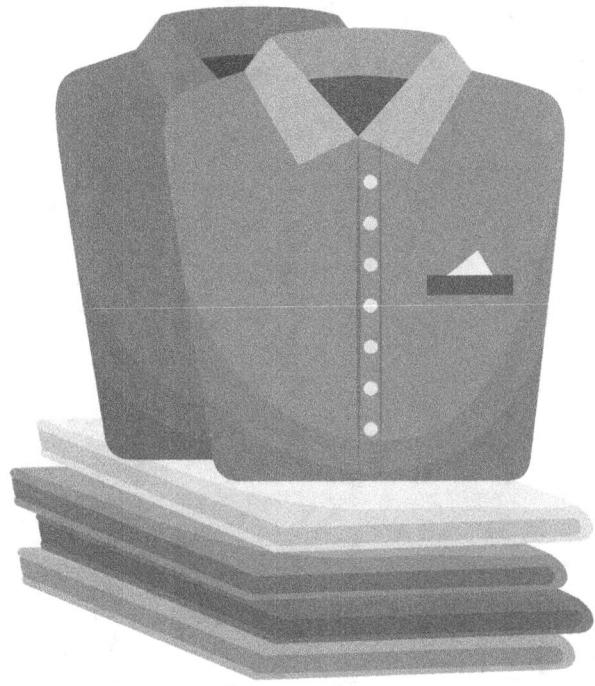

Tell me, do you enjoy folding laundry? Let me explain: It is a terrific way to keep you busy and give yourself a sense of purpose and organization.

- The folding of soft cloths and repeated actions can be relaxing.
- Classic detergent scents may stimulate pleasant memories for you.
- Folding laundry keeps you busy.

You can start with easy articles such as towels, handkerchiefs and T-shirts that are handy to fold.

Remember my dears!

It doesn't count how nicely or badly the laundry is folded, and your family members will be happy to witness you occupied and active.

Dear seniors carefully review the following pictures of different shirts and learn to fold.

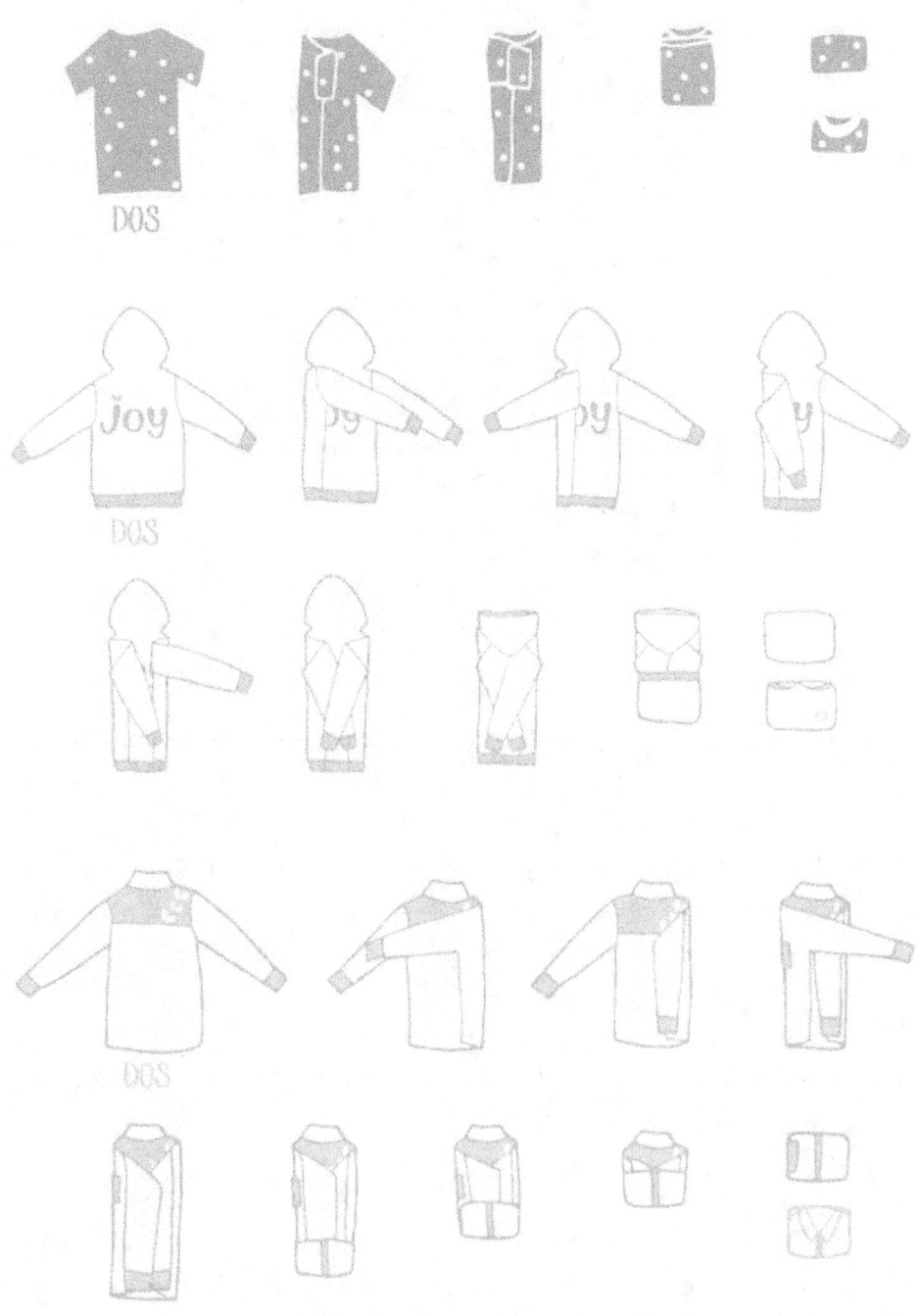

2.3. Pet Therapy

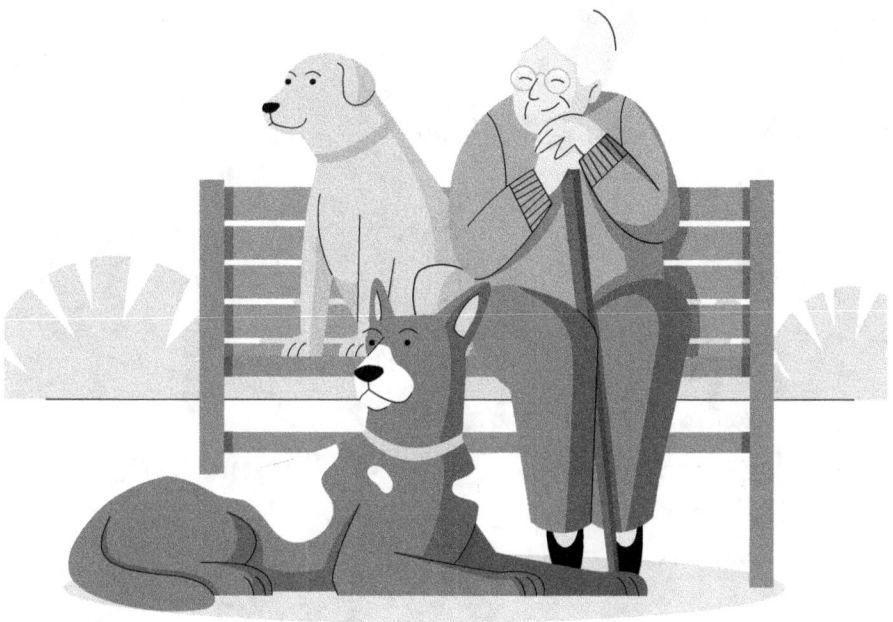

Having an animal as a pet can be calming and relaxing for many of you. Over time, it has been revealed that pets improve the quality of life of individuals, particularly seniors. Animals are not judgmental, nor are they critics of your actions. On this basis, they make an excellent partner for you with dementia. It's expected for some of you to form unique bonds with animals during therapy sessions. Occasionally, it seems that animals understand when a particular person requires some extra concentration.

Other than friendship, absolute love, and joy, animals can assist in decreasing the effects of dementia, including:

- Anxiety
- Madness
- Crankiness
- Depression
- Loneliness

Following are some of the benefits of having a pet.

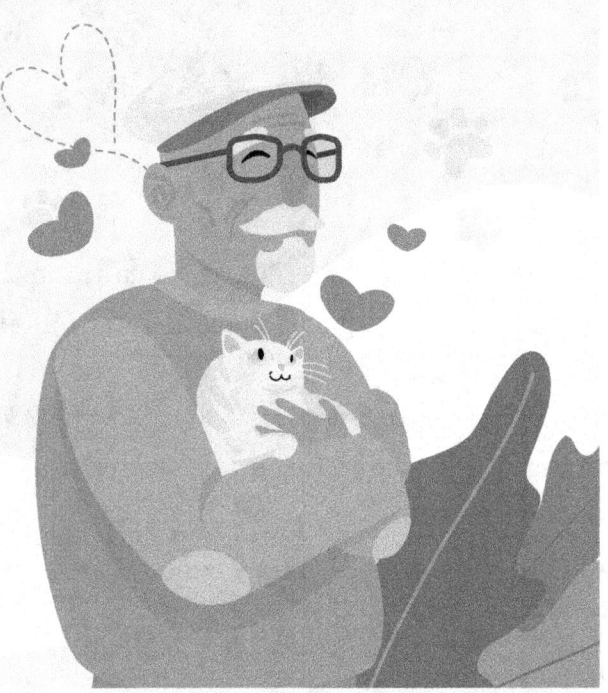

BENEFITS OF HAVING A PET

1. Animals provide affection & comfort

2. Having a pet helps us stay more active

3. Animals help reduce blood pressure

4. Pets help us socialize and meet new people

5. Animals reduce the risk of illness

2.4. Mindfulness Break

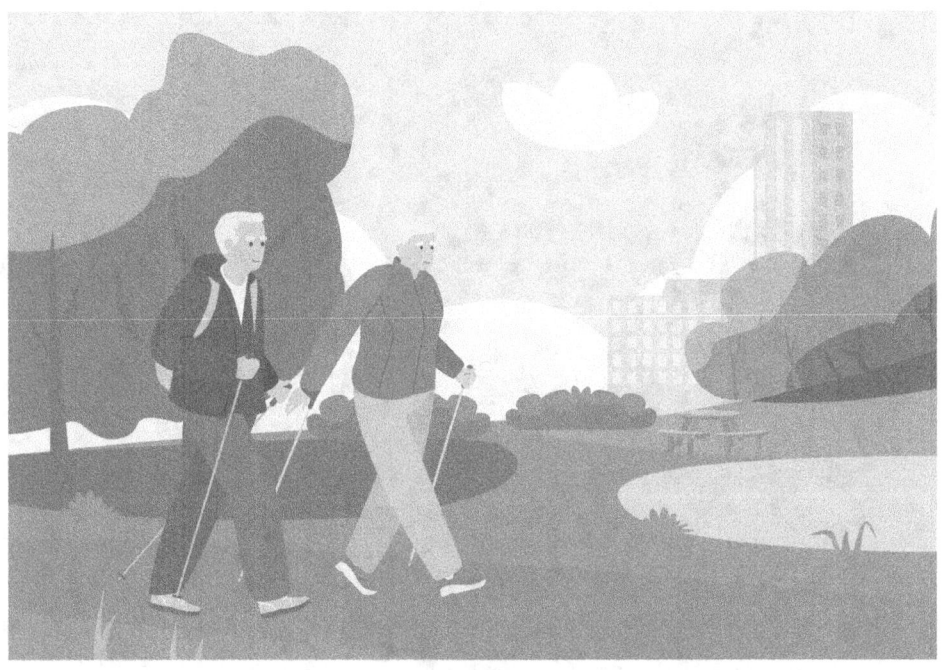

It's human instinct to appreciate the natural environment. Having a morning walk in a nearby park is always relaxing and calming to enjoy birds chirping and breathing fresh air. It's a very convenient way to meditate. Count trees or any other prominent natural object to develop deep concentration. Just to relax more, you can play with the kids or talk to them in a park. It will make you happy.

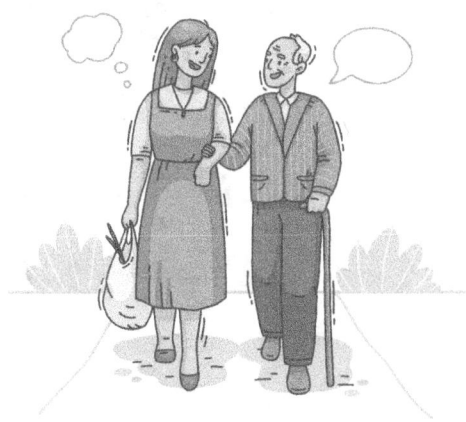

Bonus Brain Games

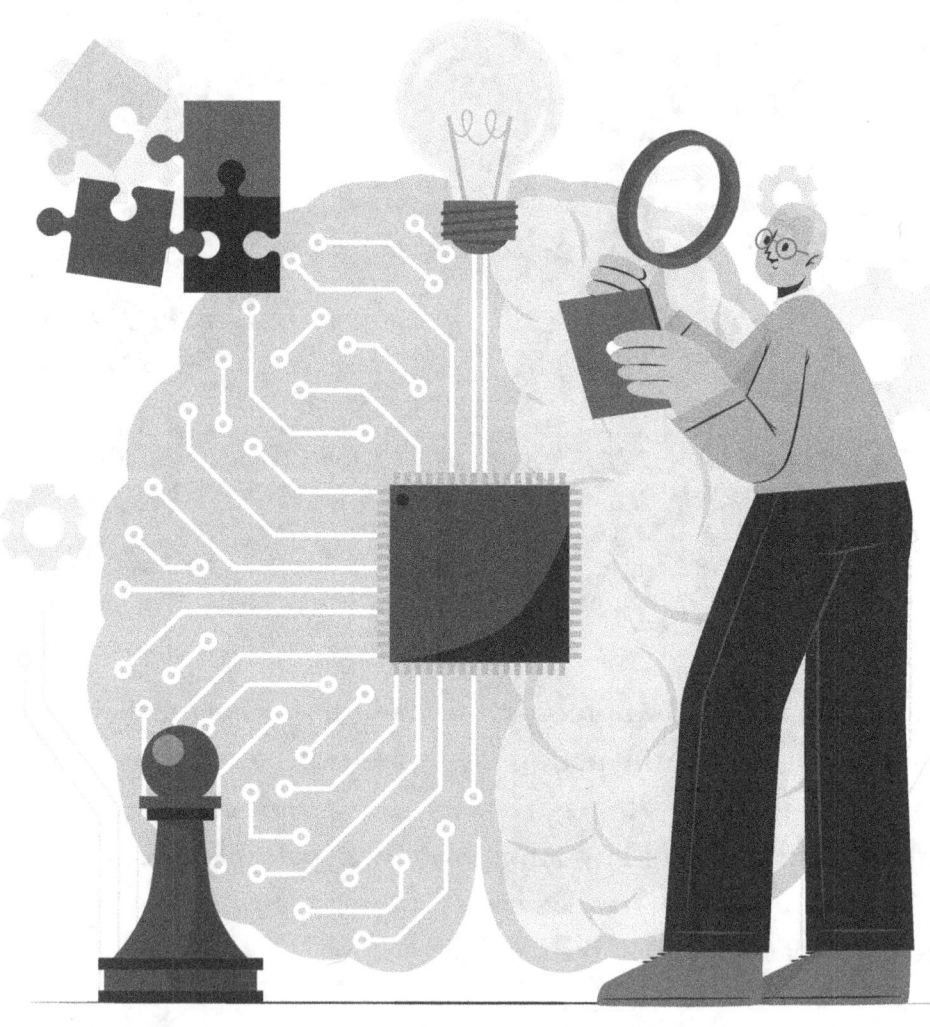

◆ **Picture Match**

INSTRUCTIONS:

In this worksheet, you must match the other half of the clothes.

MATCH THE CLOTHES

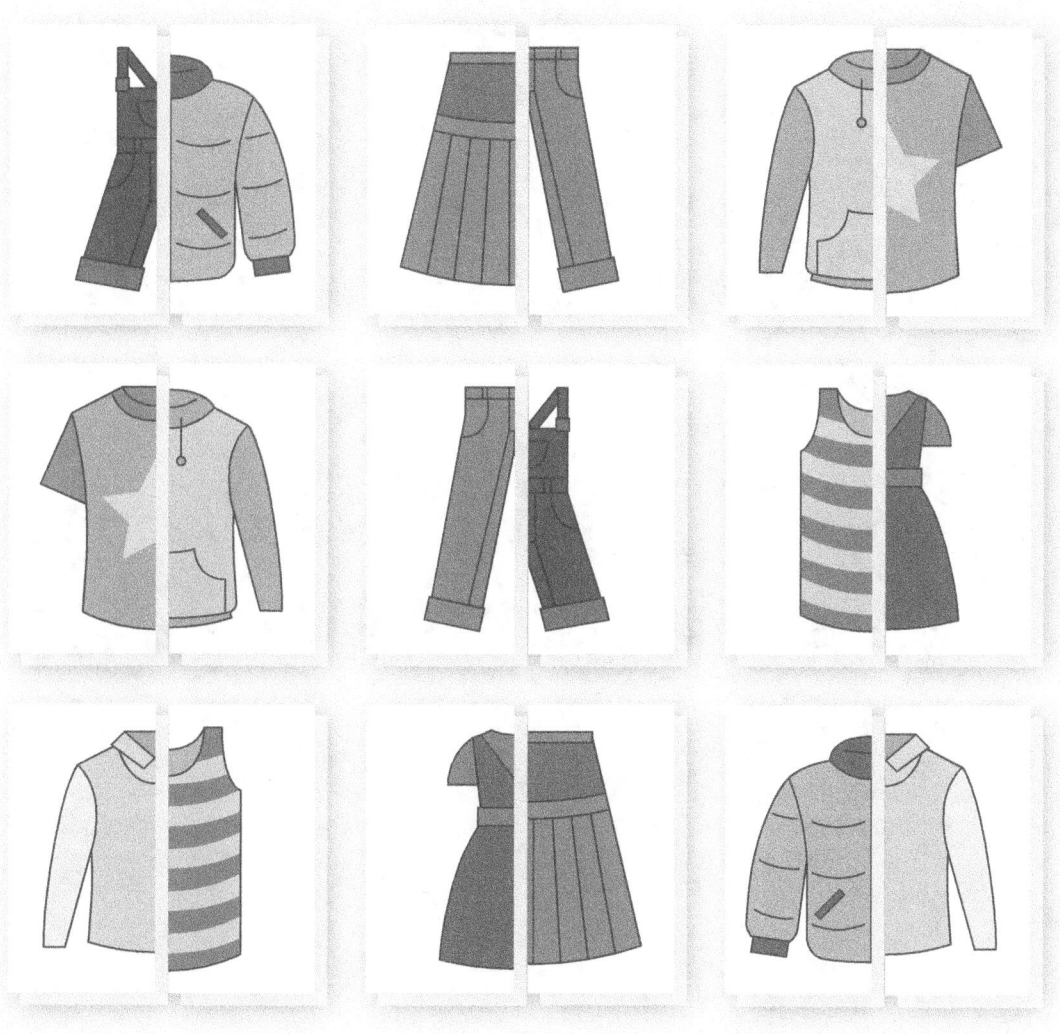

LONESOME SUSHI

In the following worksheet, most sushi pictures have at least one copy.
Find an image that has no copy or match.

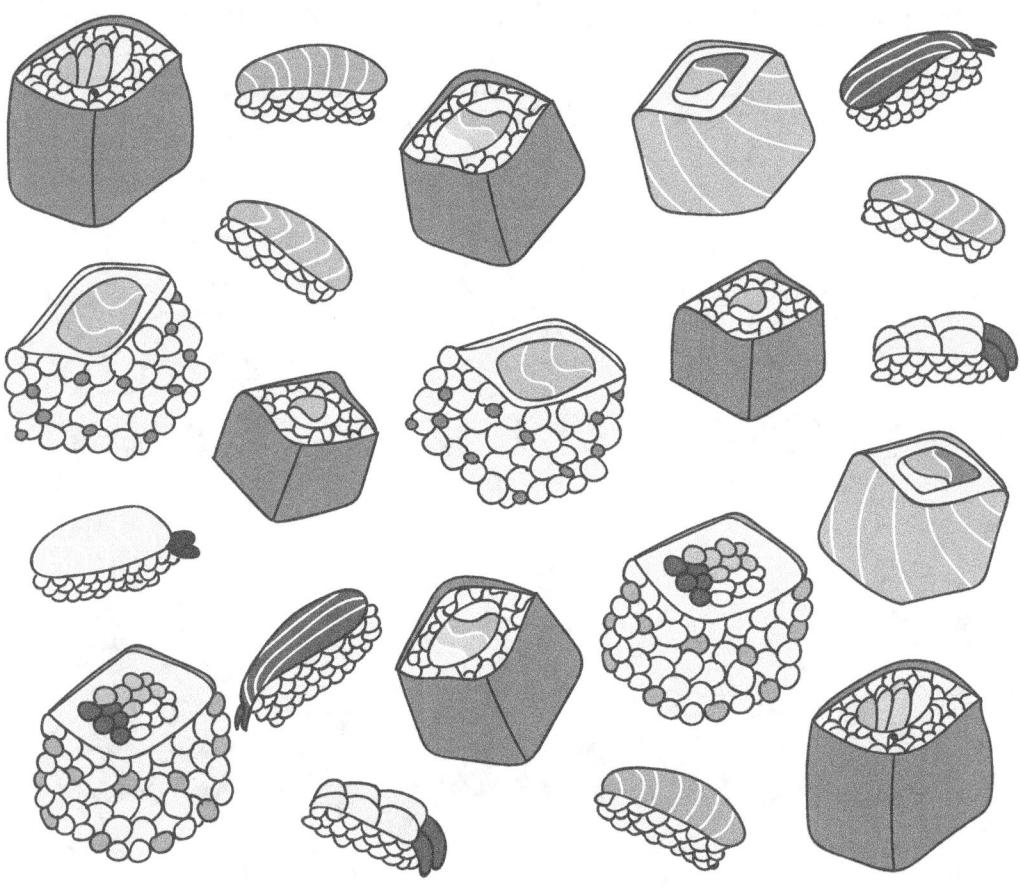

Spelling Word Scramble

Use the letters to spell the word.

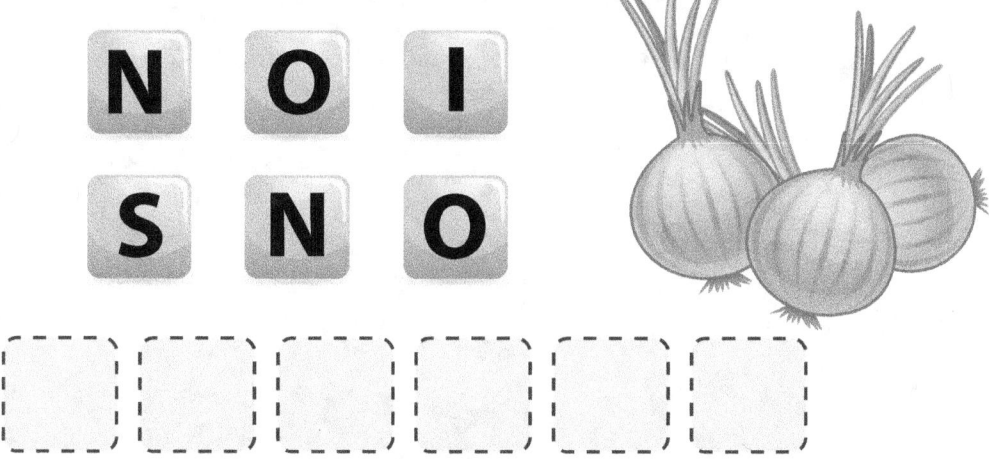

N O I

S N O

⬜ ⬜ ⬜ ⬜ ⬜ ⬜

Spelling Word Scramble

Use the letters to spell the word.

A L A

D S

⬜ ⬜ ⬜ ⬜ ⬜

MISSING DESSERT

Which sweet is missing?

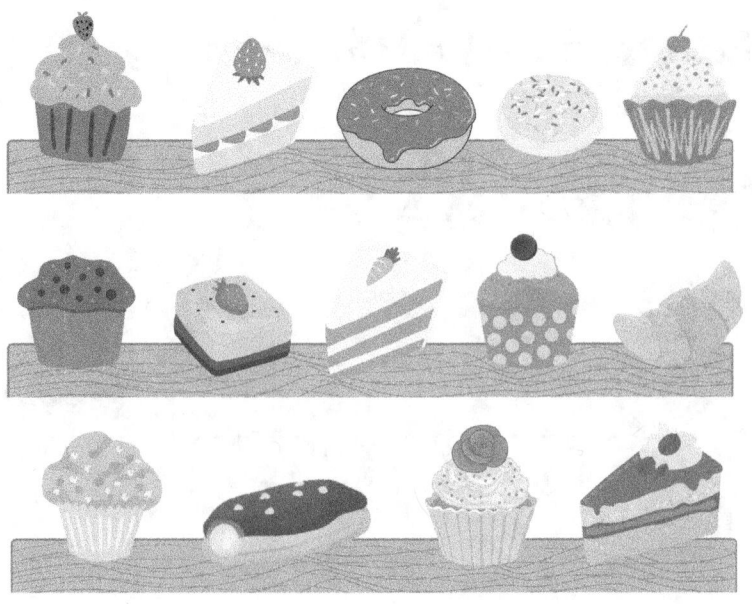

Let's do the following worksheet and complete the puzzle successfully.

FINISH THE PUZZLE

Which snap 1 - 6 finishes the puzzle?

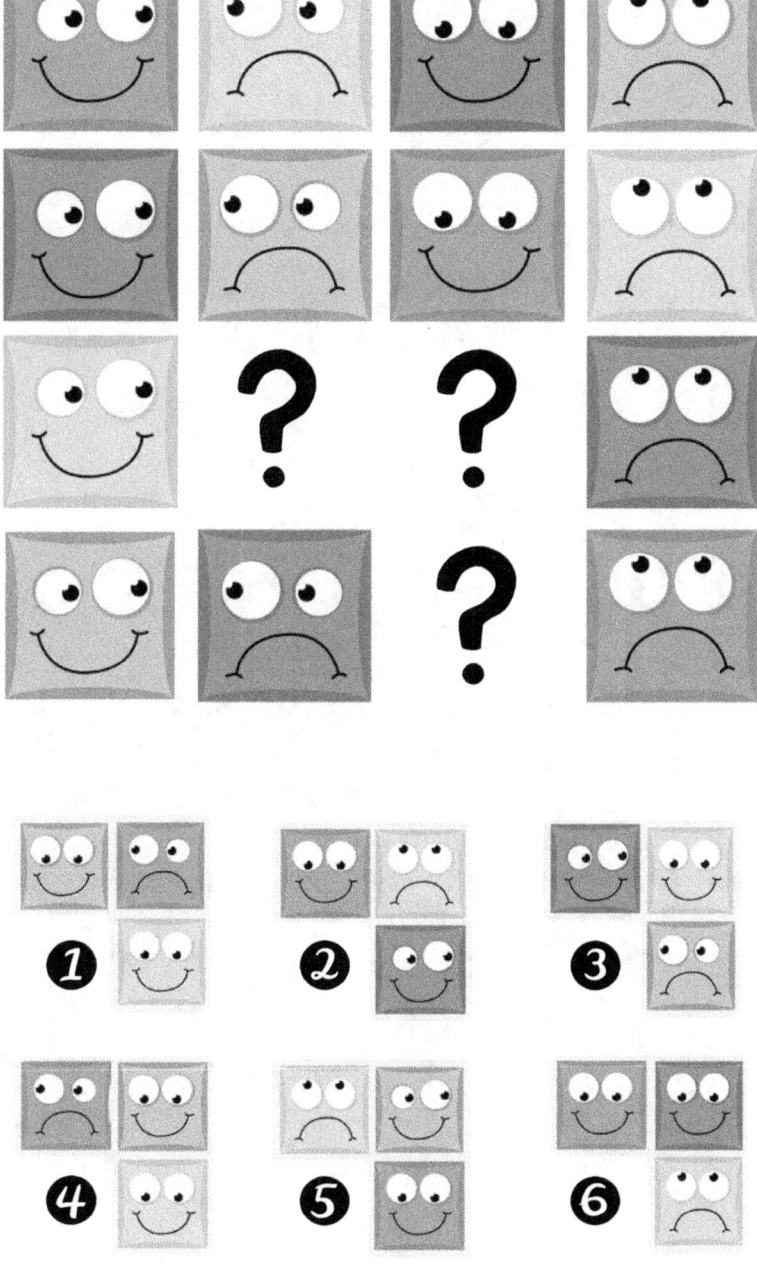

UNLOCKING THE DOOR

The key opens only one door. Can you pass this maze and open the right door?

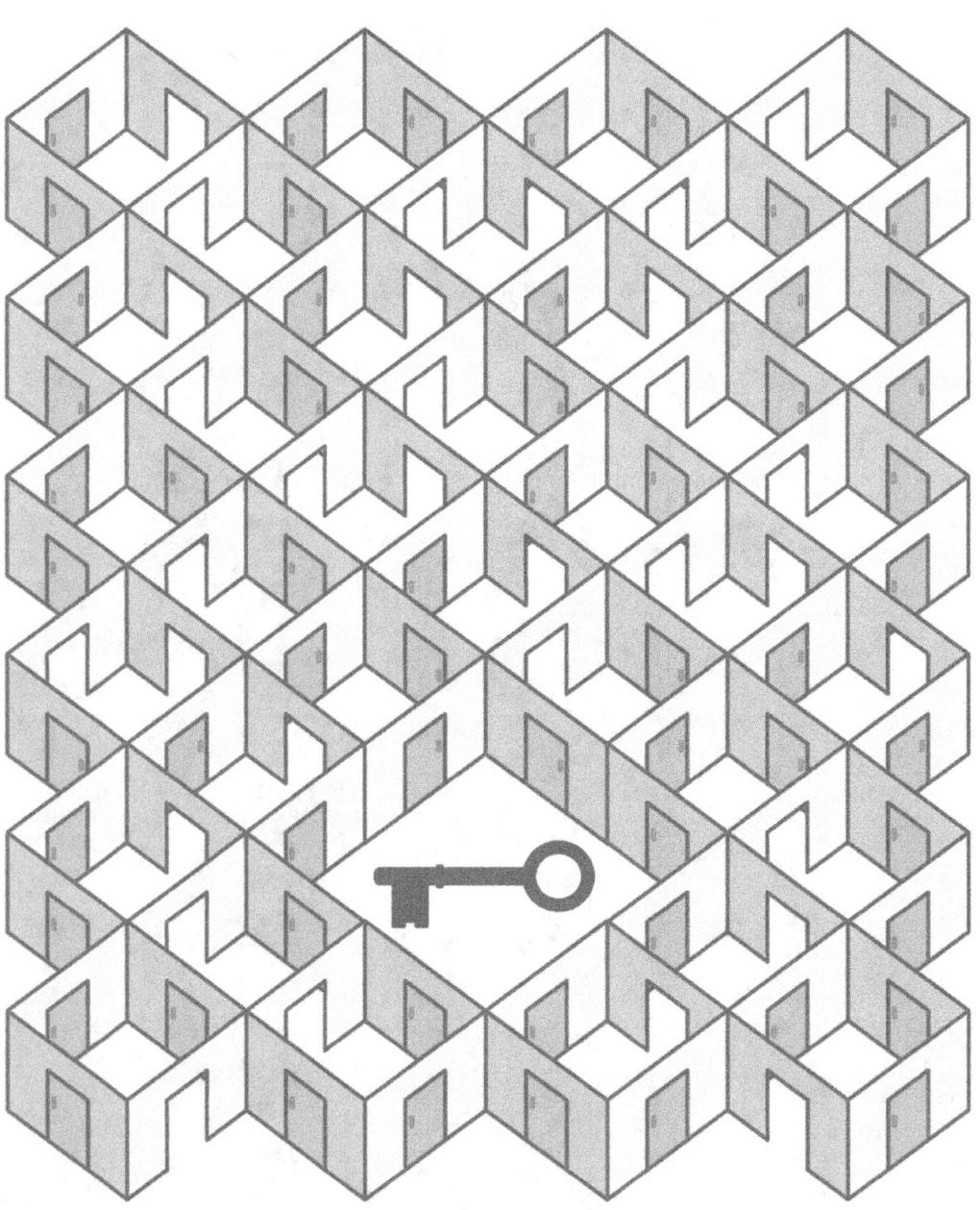

AUTUMN SEASON MAZE

Find your way through the autumn maze.

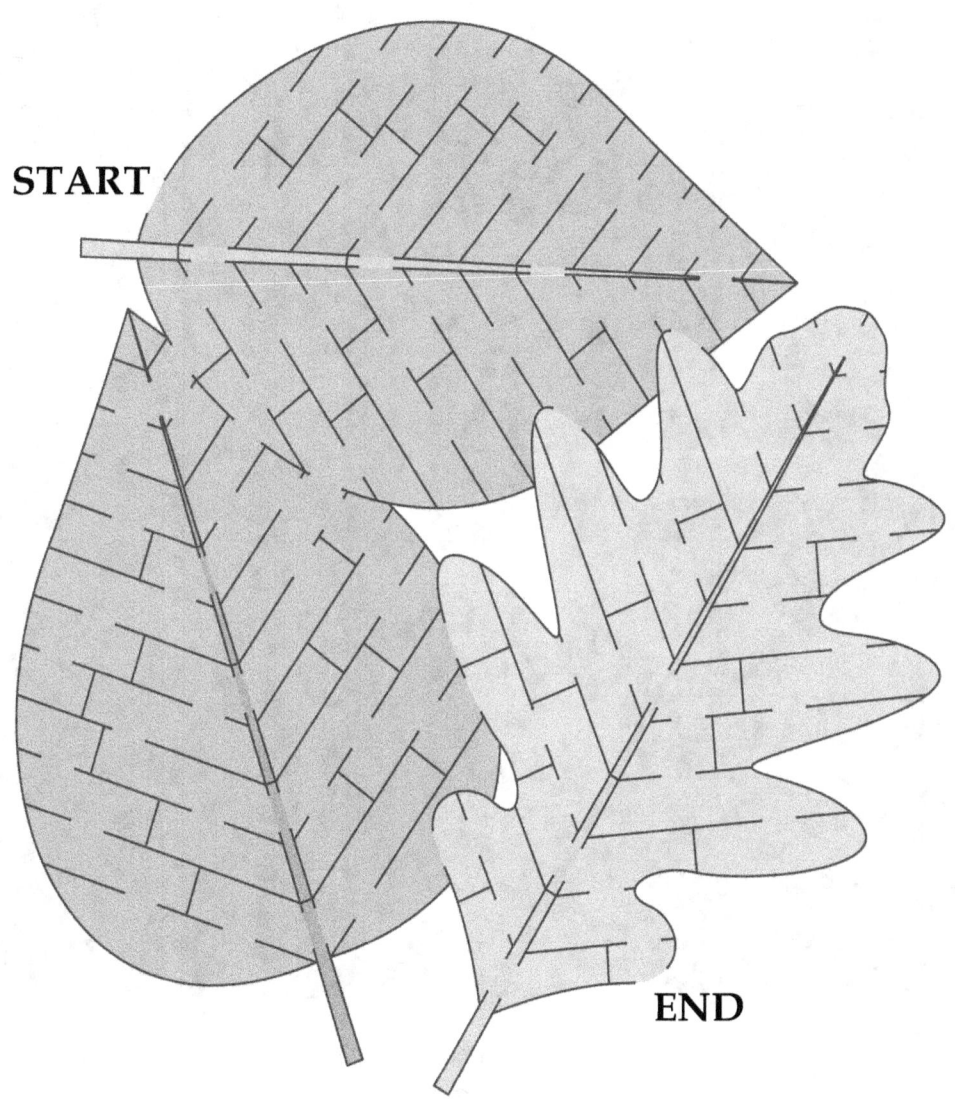

START

END

◆ **Crossword**

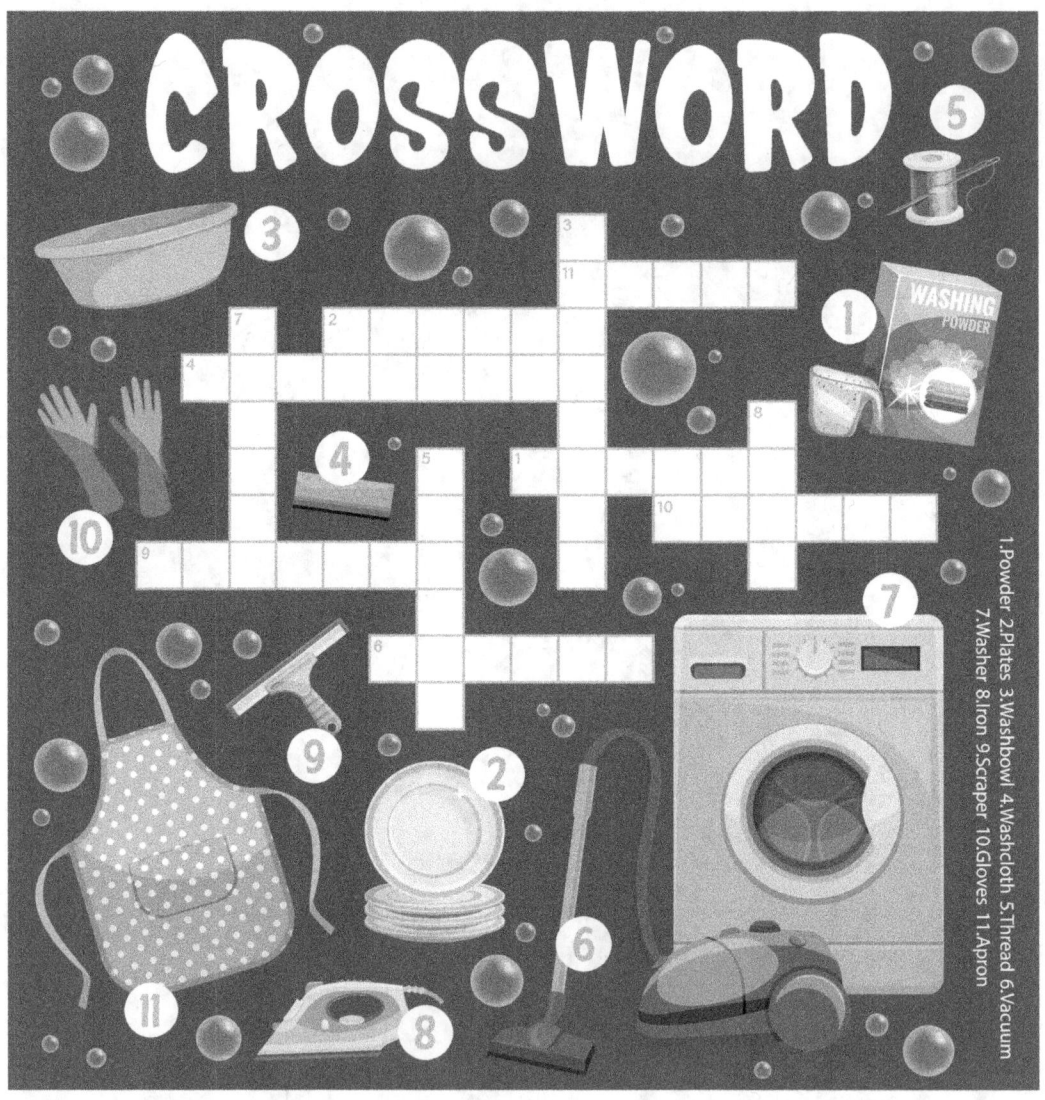

CROSSWORD

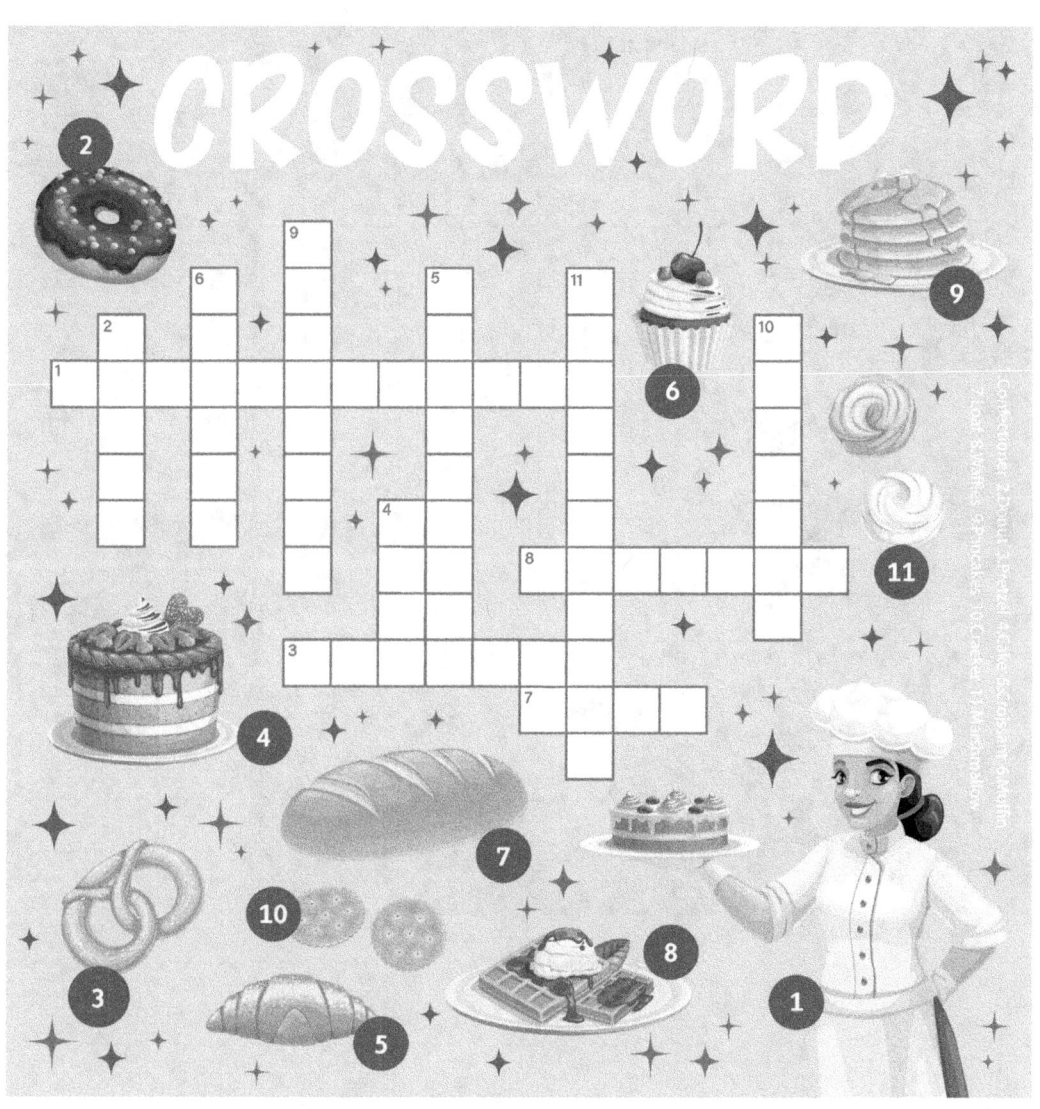

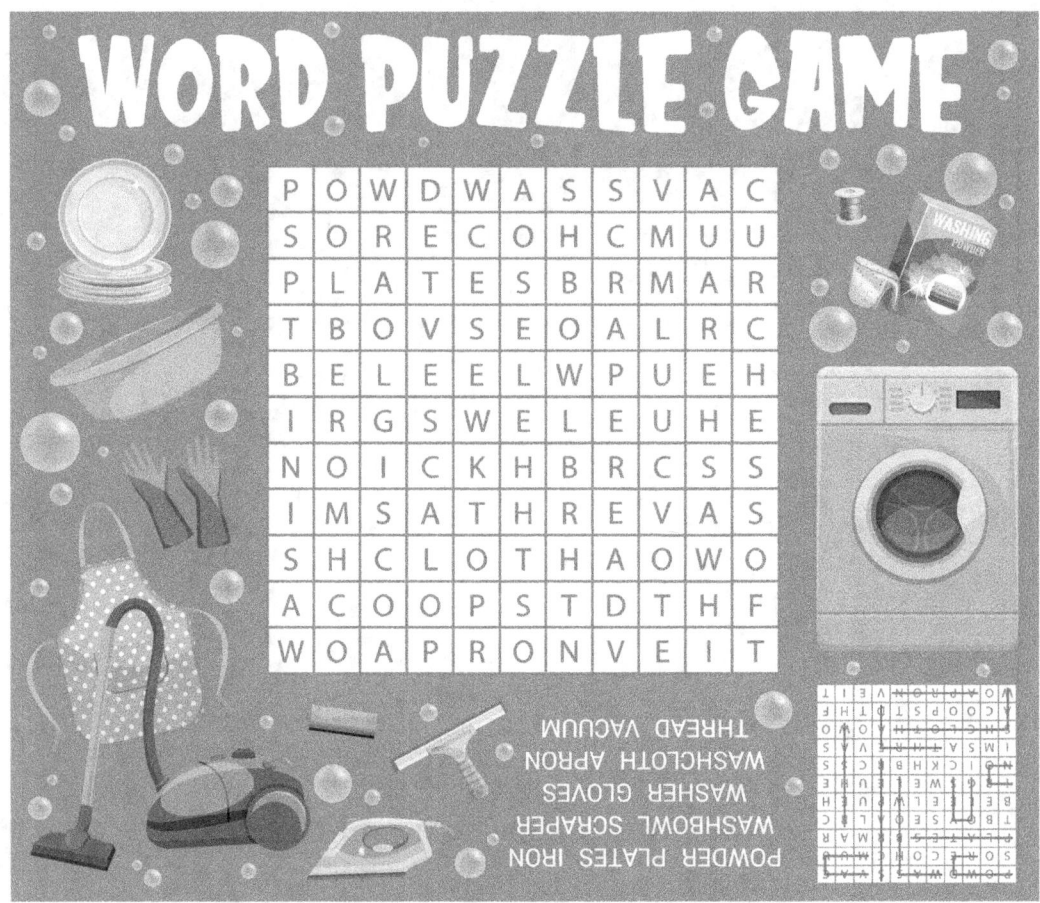

WORD PUZZLE GAME

P	O	W	D	W	A	S	S	V	A	C
S	O	R	E	C	O	H	C	M	U	U
P	L	A	T	E	S	B	R	M	A	R
T	B	O	V	S	E	O	A	L	R	C
B	E	L	E	E	L	W	P	U	E	H
I	R	G	S	W	E	L	E	U	H	E
N	O	I	C	K	H	B	R	C	S	S
I	M	S	A	T	H	R	E	V	A	S
S	H	C	L	O	T	H	A	O	W	O
A	C	O	O	P	S	T	D	T	H	F
W	O	A	P	R	O	N	V	E	I	T

POWDER PLATES IRON
WASHBOWL SCRAPER
WASHER GLOVES
WASHCLOTH APRON
THREAD VACUUM

WORD PUZZLE GAME

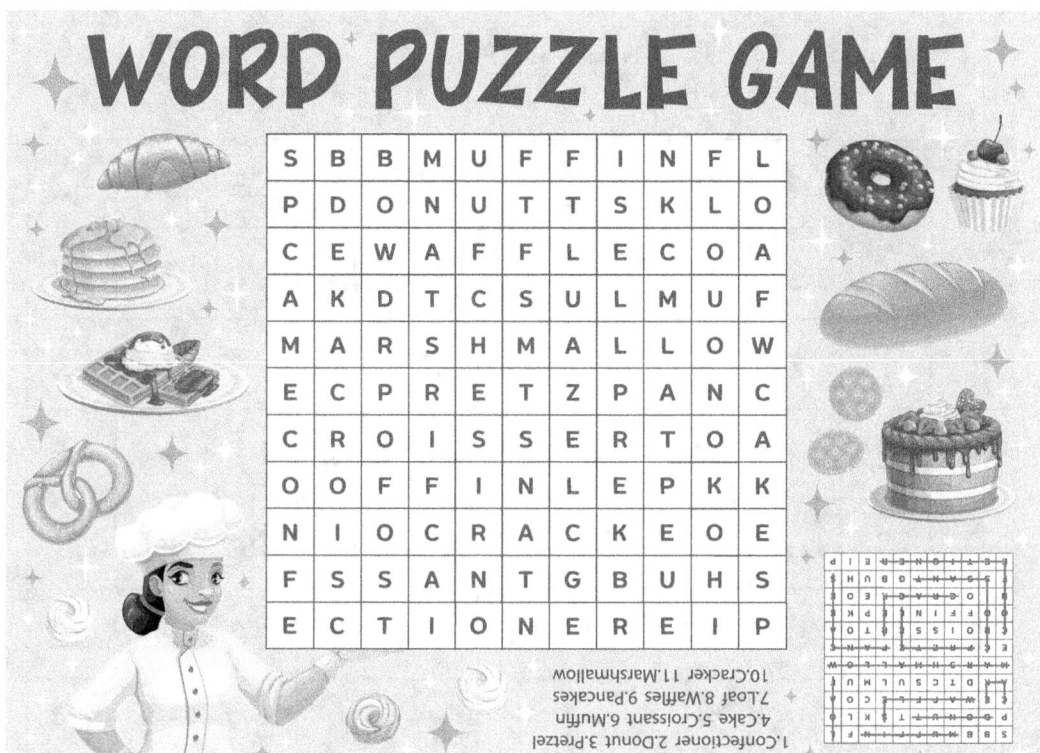

S	B	B	M	U	F	F	I	N	F	L
P	D	O	N	U	T	T	S	K	L	O
C	E	W	A	F	F	L	E	C	O	A
A	K	D	T	C	S	U	L	M	U	F
M	A	R	S	H	M	A	L	L	O	W
E	C	P	R	E	T	Z	P	A	N	C
C	R	O	I	S	S	E	R	T	O	A
O	O	F	F	I	N	L	E	P	K	K
N	I	O	C	R	A	C	K	E	O	E
F	S	S	A	N	T	G	B	U	H	S
E	C	T	I	O	N	E	R	E	I	P

1.Confectioner 2.Donut 3.Pretzel
4.Cake 5.Croissant 6.Muffin
7.Loaf 8.Waffles 9.Pancakes
10.Cracker 11.Marshmallow

TRACK NUMBERS 1 TO 55

		4	9	6	18	17	16	35	34	32
		3	8	5	20	40	15	21	23	45
1	1	2	3	4	21	23	18	20	30	46
3	2	9	8	13	12	31	30	19	48	47
9	3	6	7	8	20	12	17	18	19	31
8	4	5	22	9	10	11	16	40	20	32
10	5	26	23	10	42	41	15	39	21	33
14	6	25	24	11	12	13	14	39	22	47
8	7	14	15	16	17	18	19	20	23	46
21	34	33	32	31	40	27	26	25	24	55
23	35	18	19	30	29	28	27	28	29	54
24	36	30	32	31	5	2	50	51	52	53
38	37	38	39	46	47	48	49	44	55	54
39	20	33	44	45	29	52	53	45		
40	41	42	43	46	47	53	54	55		

TRACK THE NUMBERS

Can you find the sequence of 1 to 10?

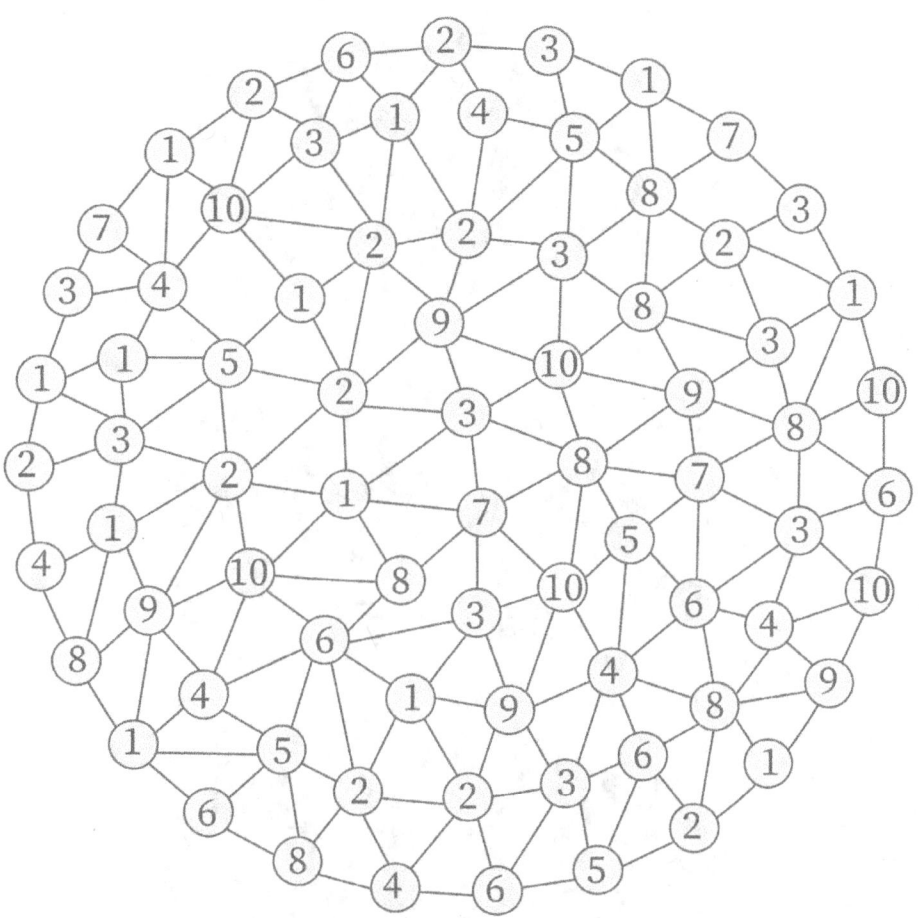

◆ Pattern Recognition

Can you recognize the missing slice of cake from 1 to 6?

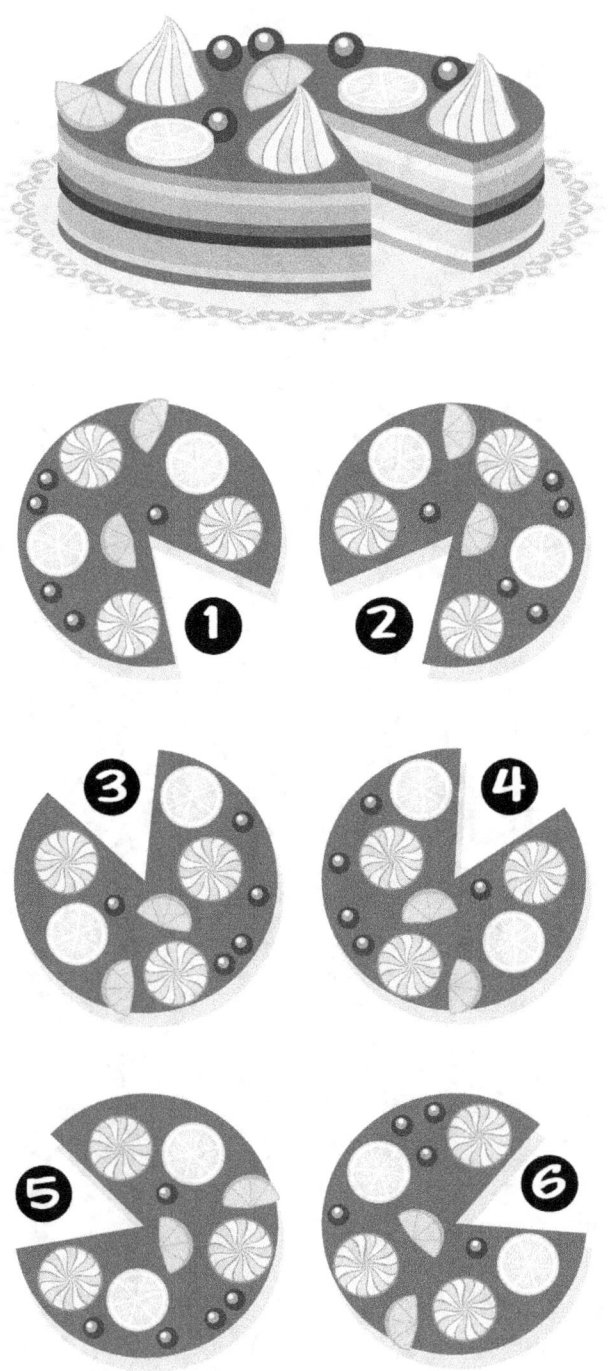

MIRROR PICTURES

Every row has a mirrored row. Can you find the mirror pictures in each row?

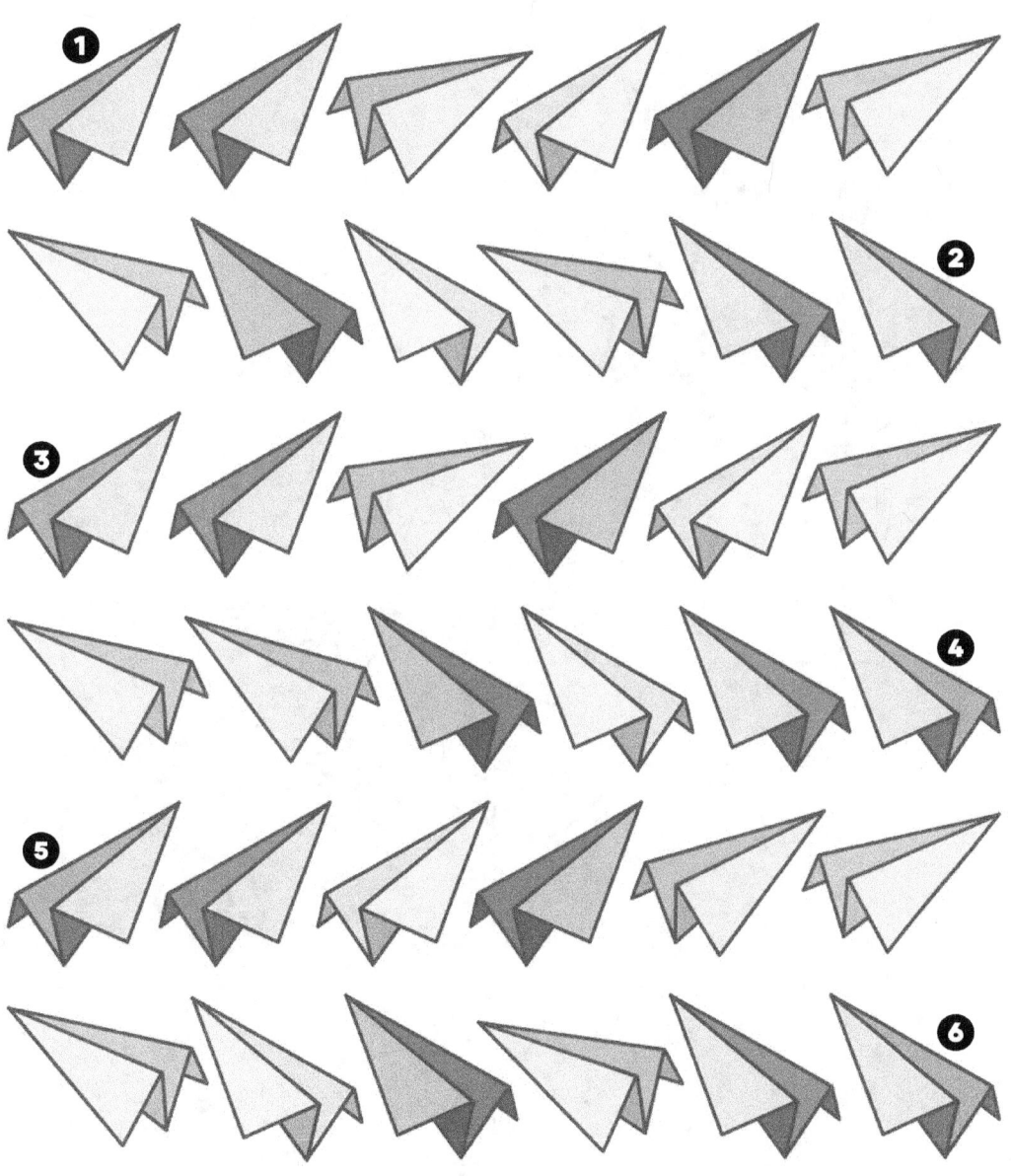

CAN YOU IDENTIFY 8 DIFFERENCES?

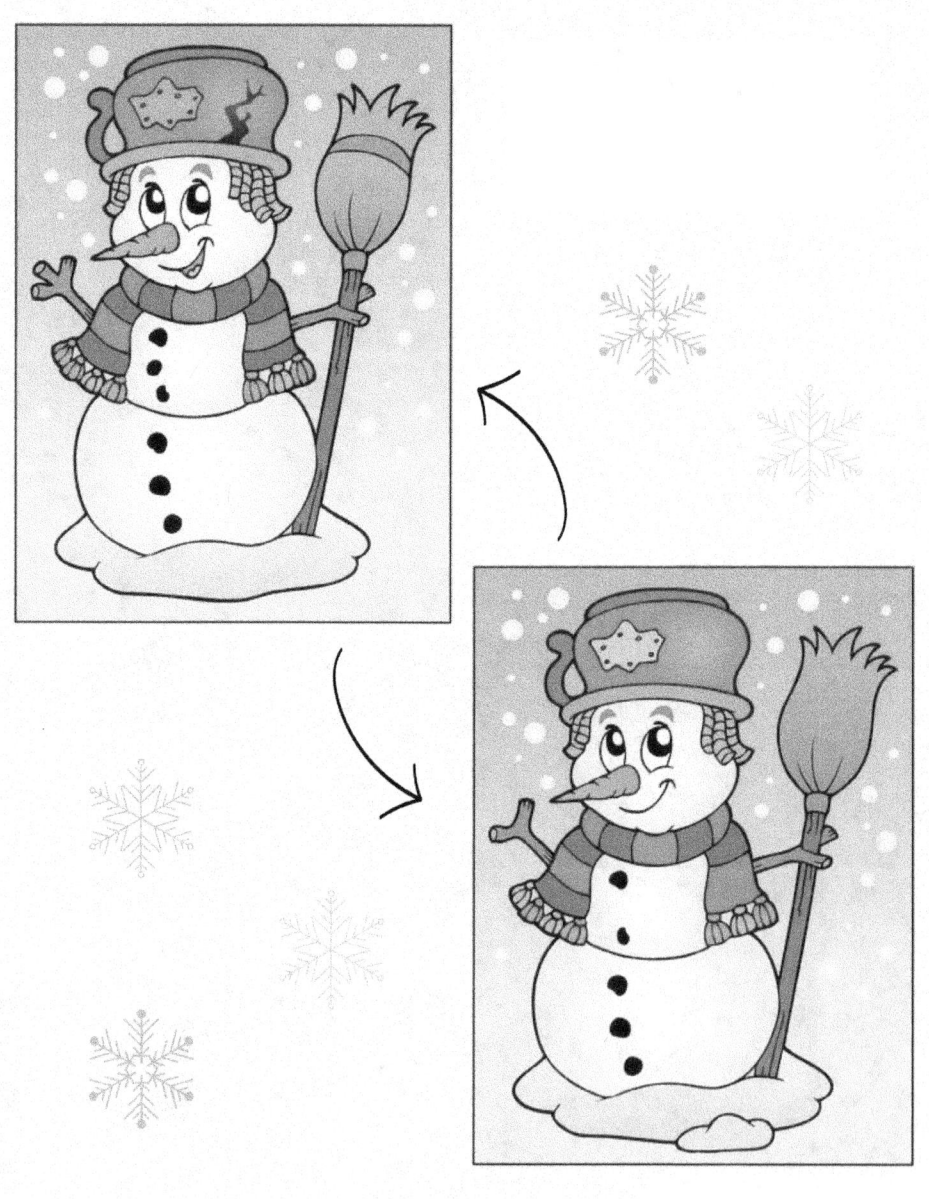

EAGLE EYES, CAN YOU SPOT 10 DIFFERENCES?

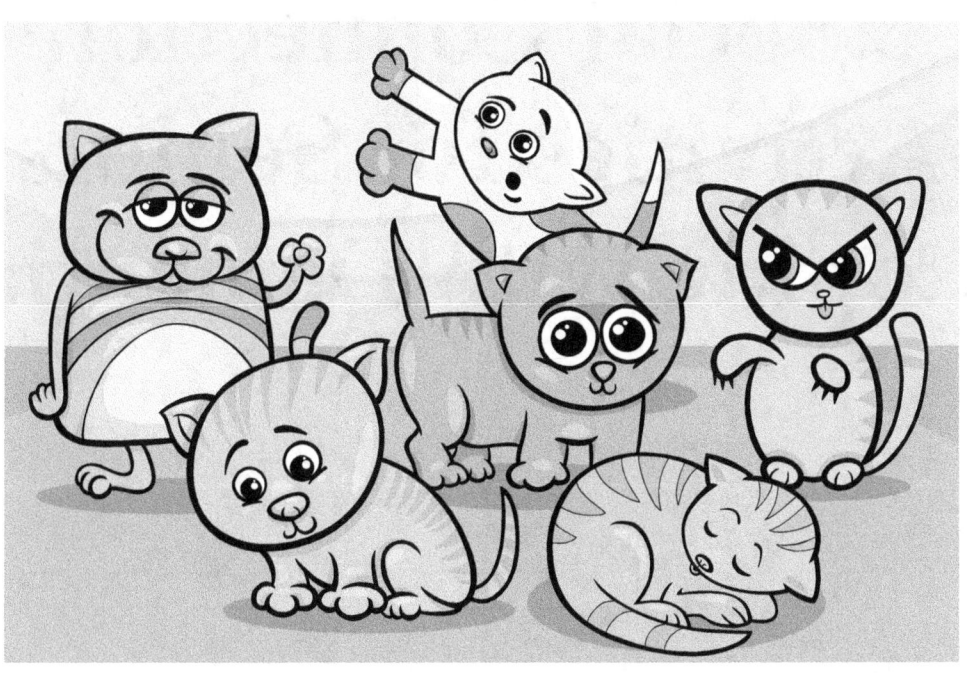

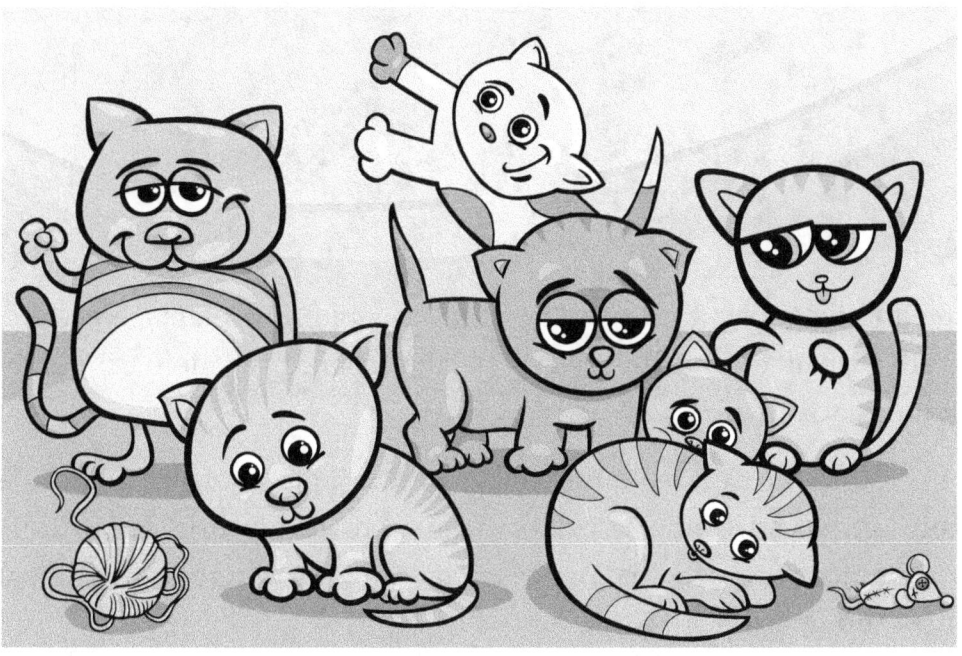

PART - III
3.Social Connection Activities for Seniors Coping with Dementia

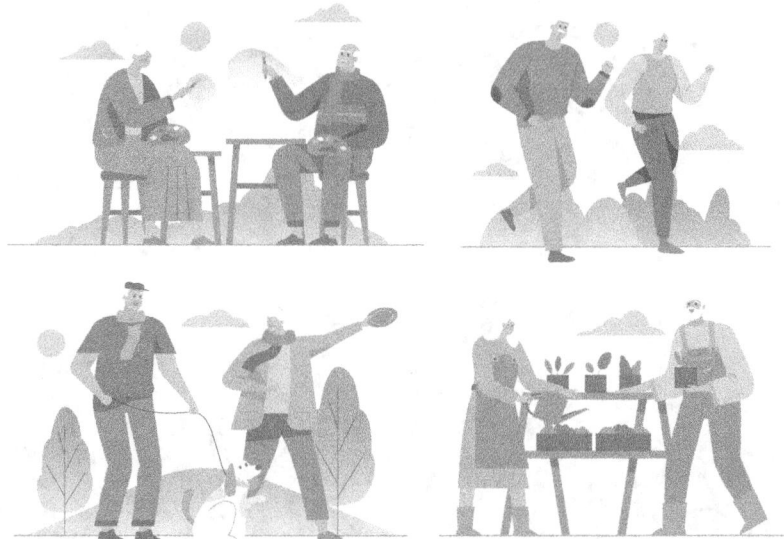

After the diagnosis of dementia, many people find themselves feeling socially isolated and deprived of the chance to deliver valuable assistance to others.

But most of you still have the ability and urge to contribute and make significant social connections; you must create meeting opportunities and community participation to socialize with others with the same values and interests.

3.1. Community Activities

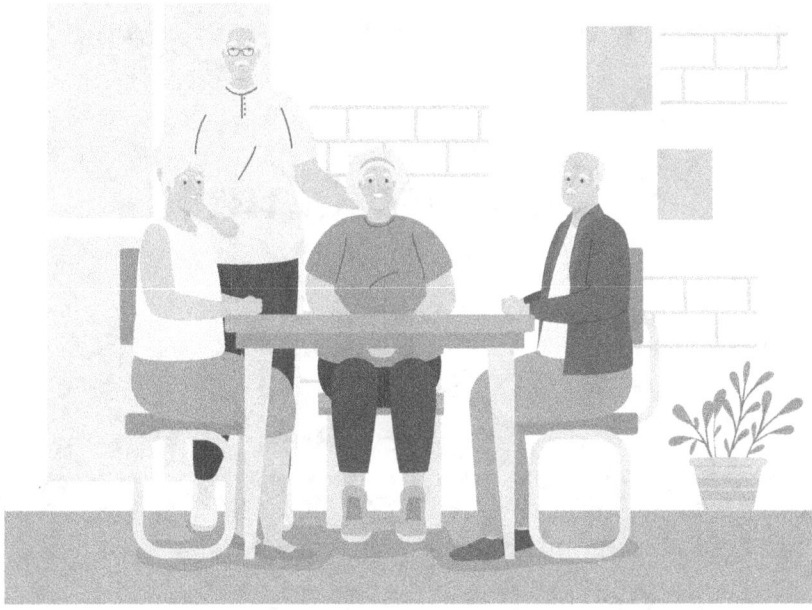

The most essential characteristic of being in a community is having the possibility for strong social connections.

- Some communities have organized programs to encourage service and participation between seniors and the residents of the community.
- Volunteering is another excellent option to engage in the local community if such programs aren't functional.

There are also some other ways to contribute to household well-being, for example:

✓ Gardening

✓ Meal preparation

✓ Table setting

✓ Dusting

You can positively influence the quality of life and health by offering small opportunities to participate in discussions with your family while assisting them in chores. You can also share your beautiful memories with your loved ones, which will help you retain memories and make connections. You can also invite your neighbors or friends to revive the memory process.

3.2. Group Games

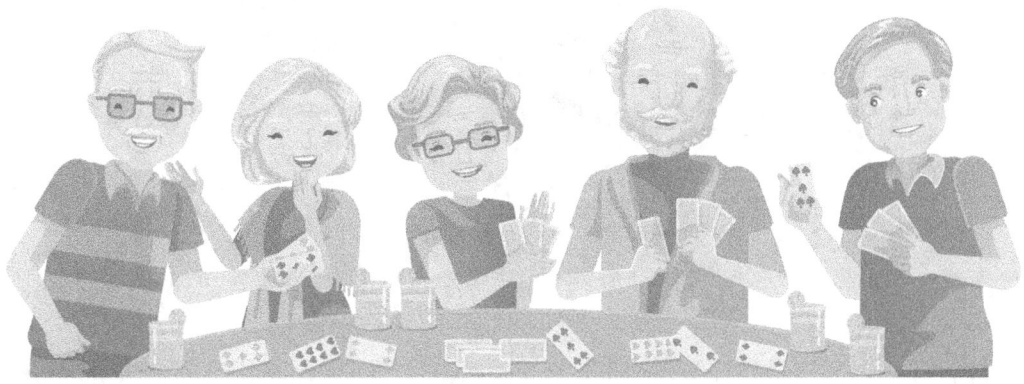

Participating in group games can promote both cognitive and social interaction. The following classic games are suggested for you:

- ✓ Dominoes
- ✓ Checkers
- ✓ Bingo
- ✓ Ludo
- ✓ Cards
- ✓ Chess

It can be an excellent choice for you. You can enjoy these board games with your grandchildren, friends or family. These games are classic and can be more straightforward than knowing the rules of a new and unfamiliar game. These games can boost memory as they help you remember how to play them and the moves you take in the game.

3.3. Outdoor Activities

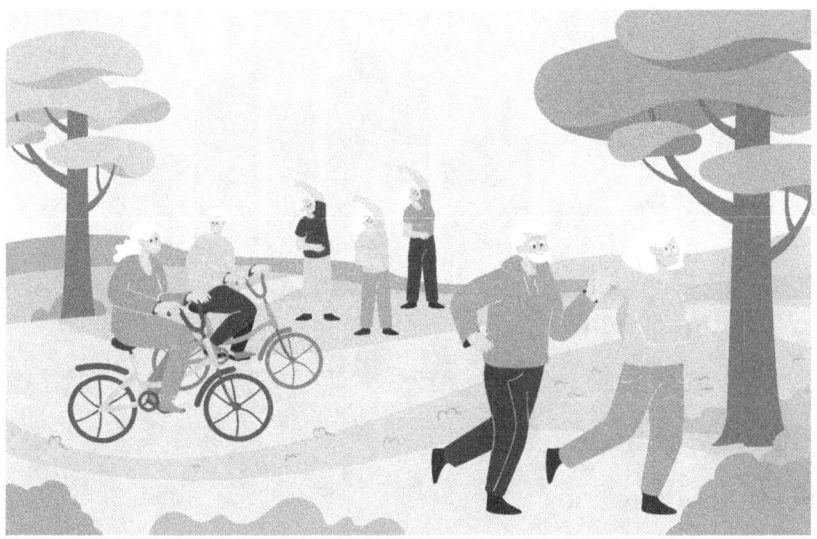

Outdoor activities on pleasant days are a fabulous way to sharpen the senses and get you active and moving.

There are numerous factors to consider when scheduling outdoor activities for yourself:

- ✓ Physical constraint
- ✓ Danger of wandering
- ✓ Conveyance
- ✓ Weather
- ✓ Seasons of year

When evaluating the season, time of year and weather, there are additional advantages of summer activities for you, such as:

- ✓ Vitamin D
- ✓ Fresh breezes
- ✓ Sunlight

The following activities have been shown to influence mood positively.

- ✓ Going for a walk
- ✓ Planting
- ✓ Feeding the birds
- ✓ Leaves raking
- ✓ Visiting the park
- ✓ Swinging on a swing
- ✓ Dogs watching at a dog park
- ✓ Catching or tossing a ball
- ✓ Playing horseshoes
- ✓ Enjoying the beach or visiting the forest
- ✓ Arranging a picnic in the lawn

Outdoor time on a lovely day doing activities like walking with fellows and family, doing some physical exercises such as yoga, reading books, or discussing political or other interests can also help you relax and memorize old days and lower levels of depression and anxiety.

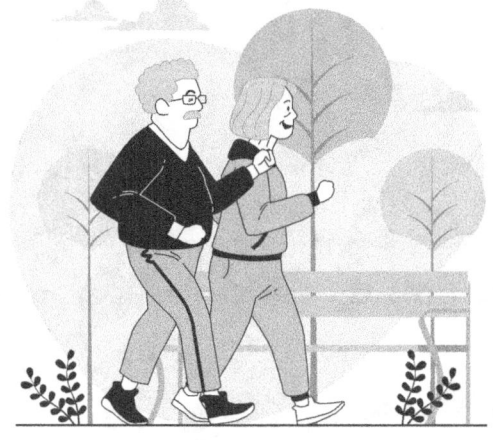

3.4. Mindfulness Break

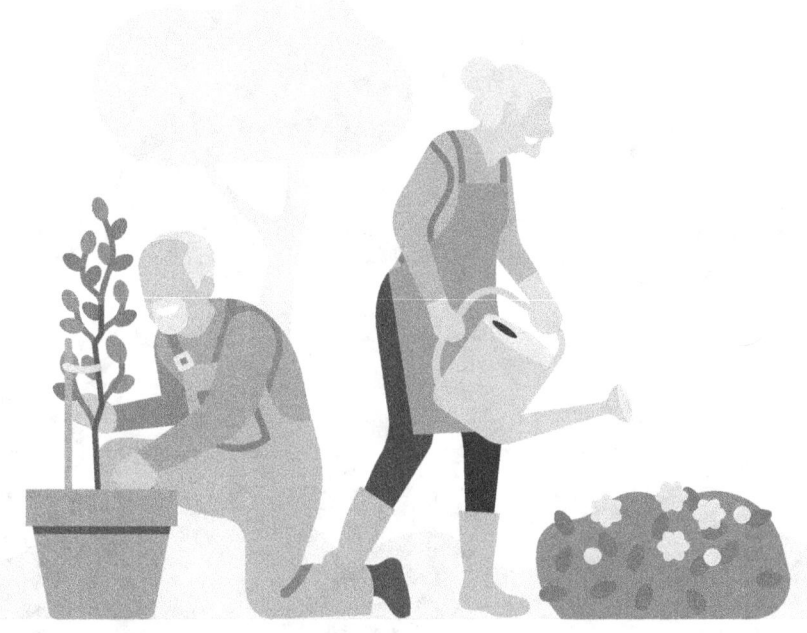

Caring for the garden or growing plants can be relaxing and healthy, especially starting with a small-sized green area. Likewise, you can concentrate on bonding with nature; inhaling and exhaling around nature helps you relax and takes you back to when you were younger, how you played in gardens, and your gossiping time with friends. You can choose aromatic plants that help reduce stress, like mint plants, and place them where you usually sit in your garden for meditation.

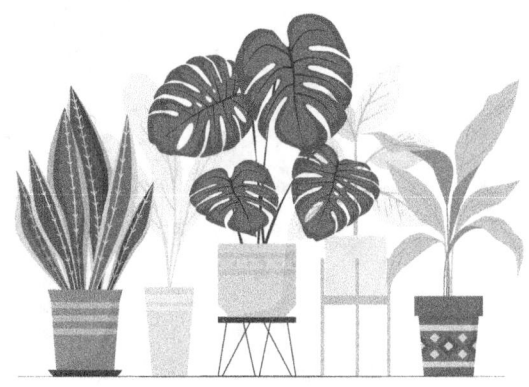

Bonus Brain Games

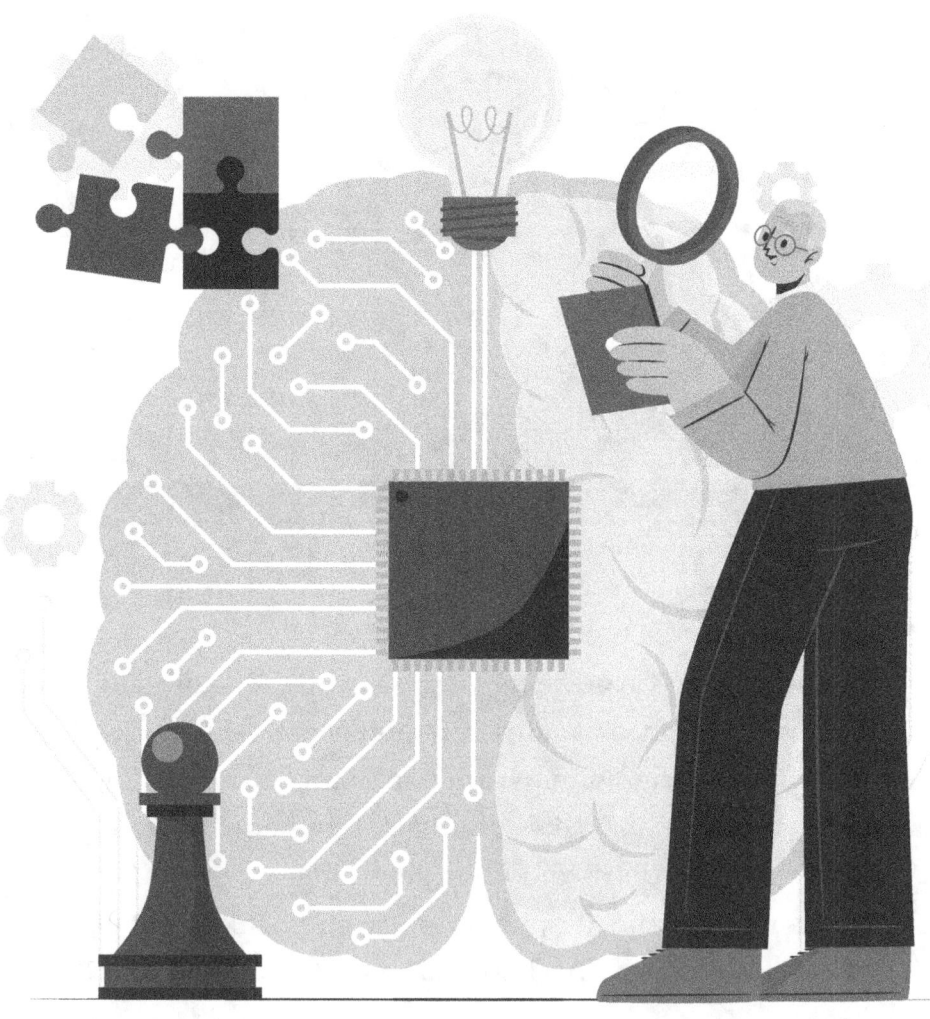

CAN YOU FIND THE MATCHING SNOWFLAKES?

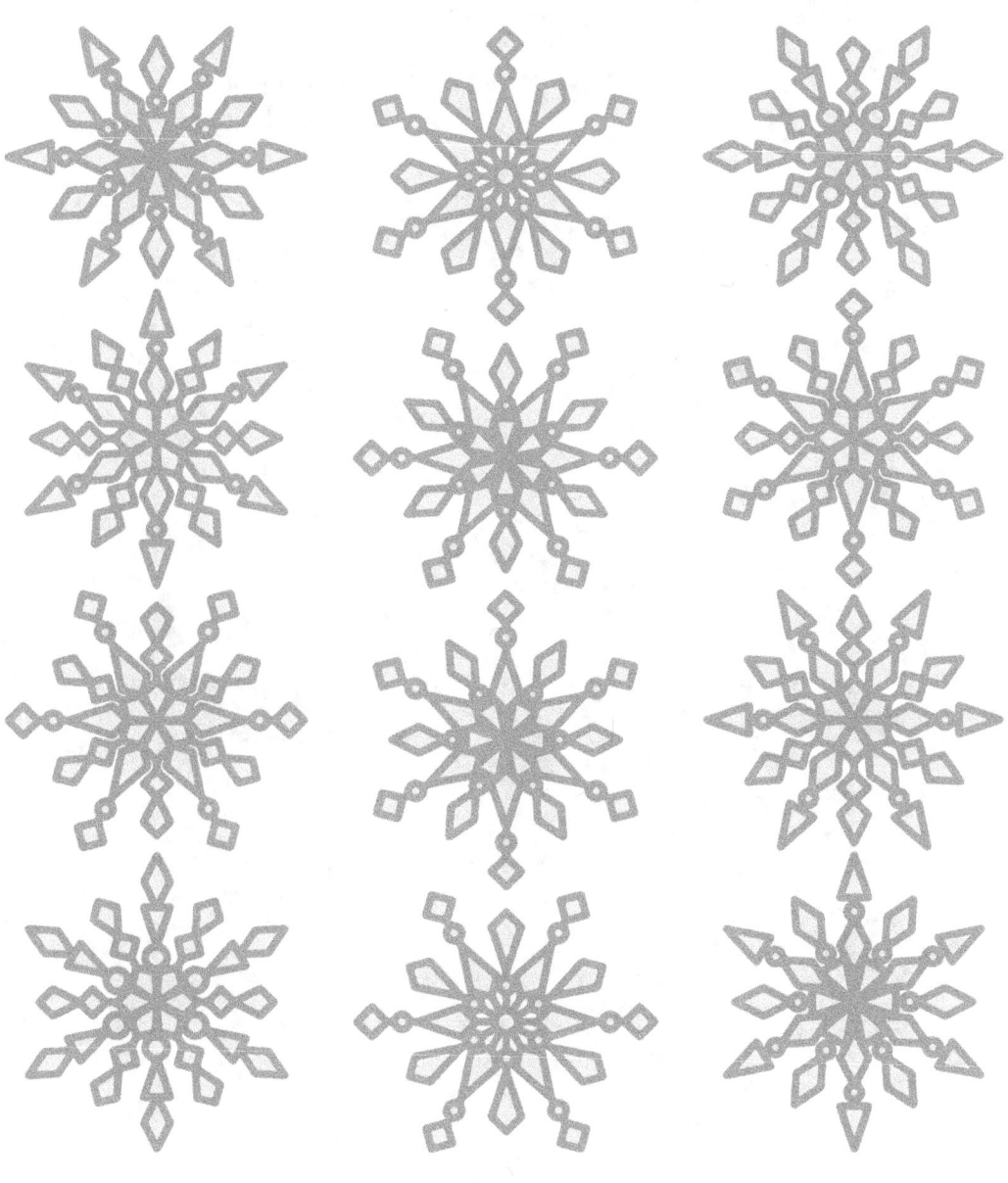

FIND THE MATCHING PAIR
OF PEAPOD

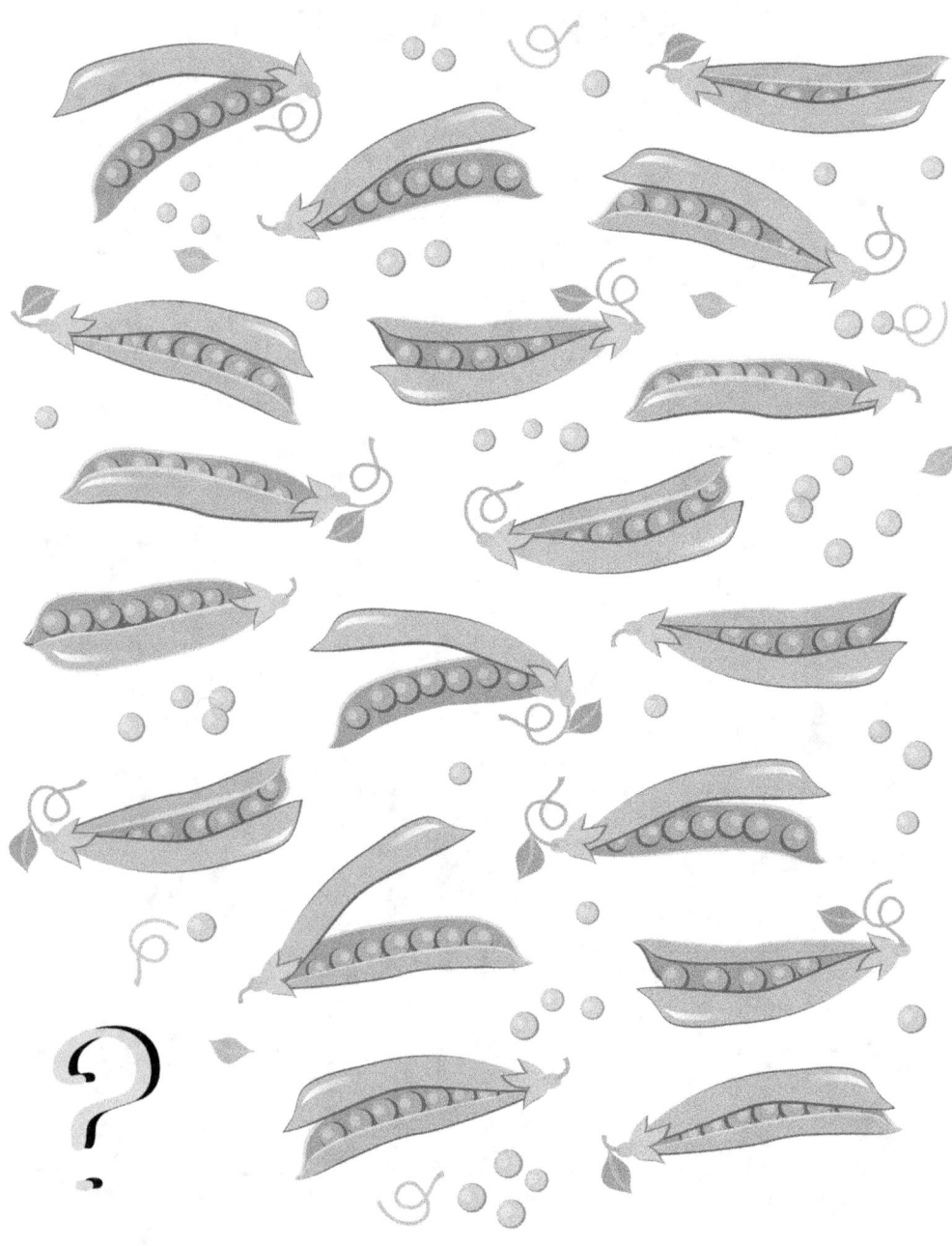

GUESS KNOT

Can you find when you pull which string will form a knot?

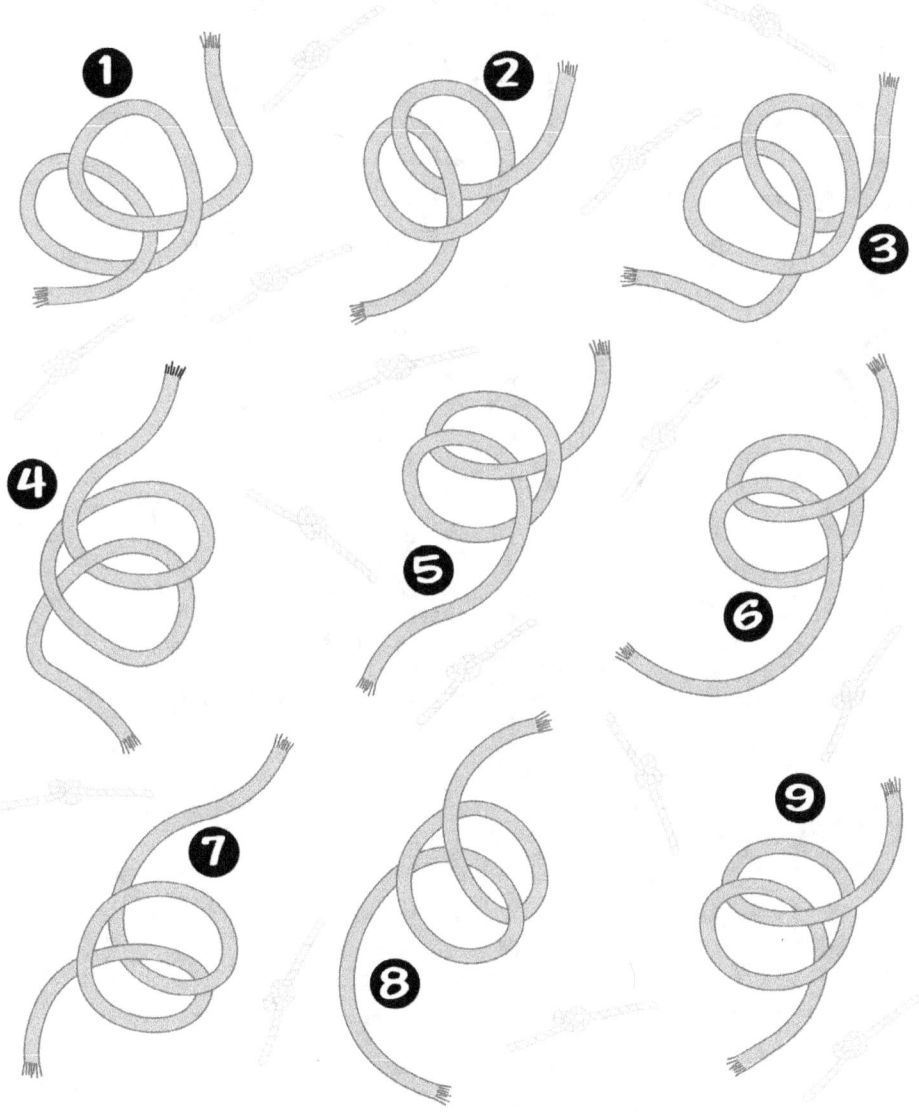

COUNTING THE SHAPES

Can you find and count the geometrical shapes?

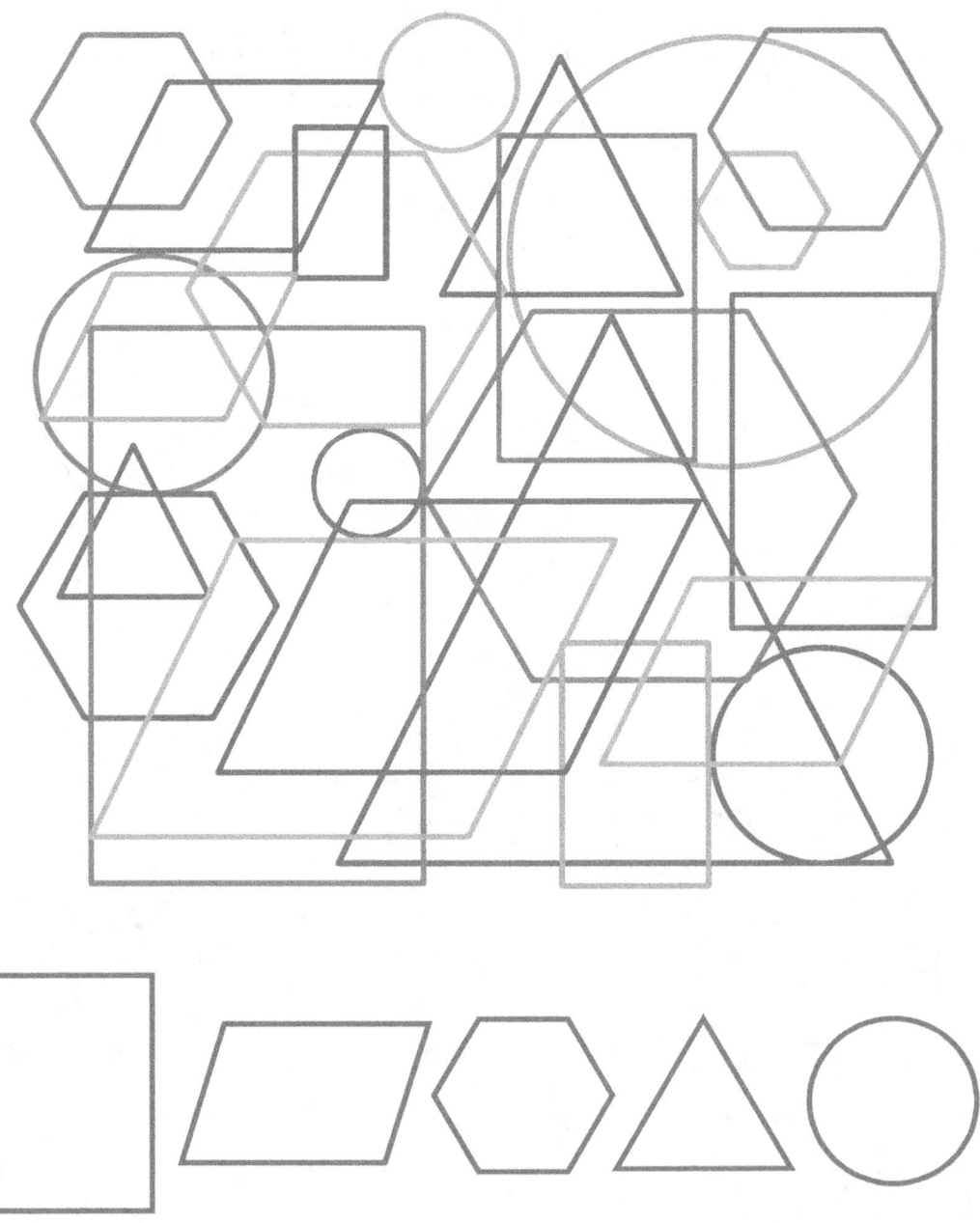

CAN YOU HELP THE COUPLE MEET?

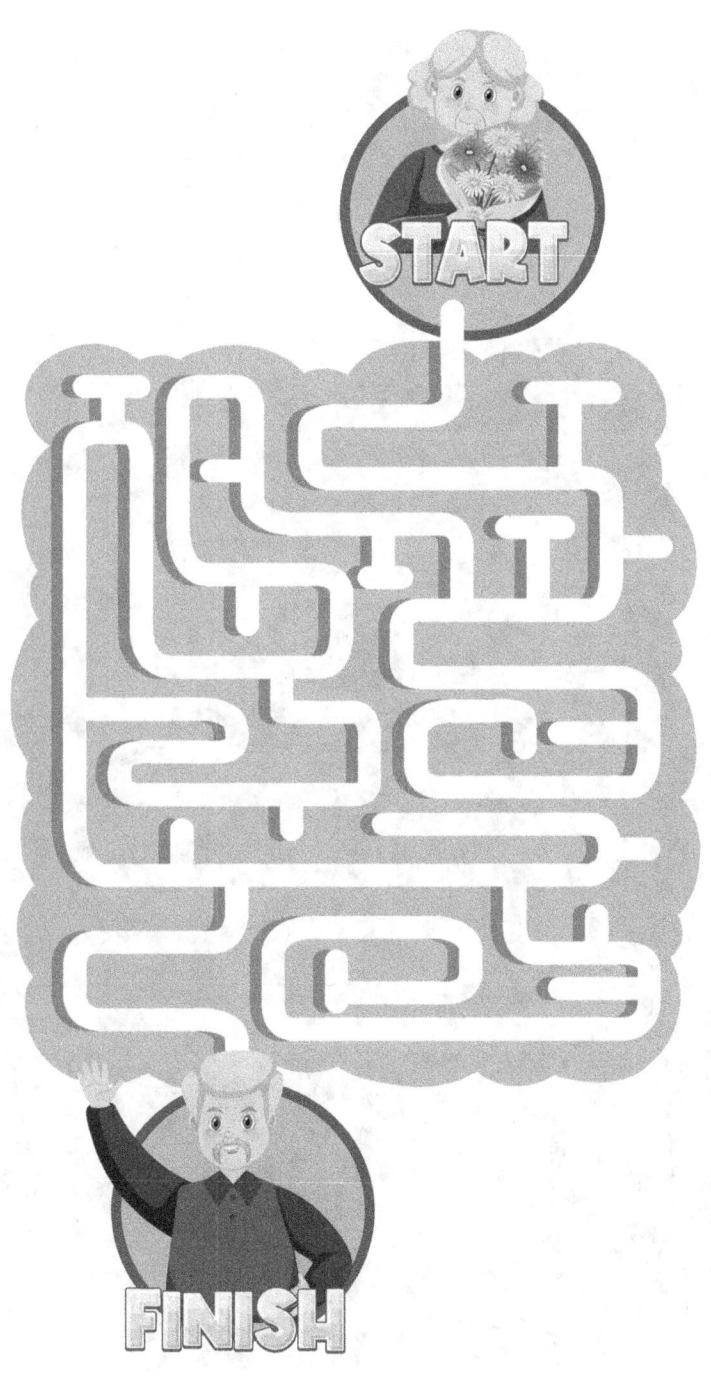

Oops, two ants are stuck in the hole. Can you help them go out and reunite with their family?

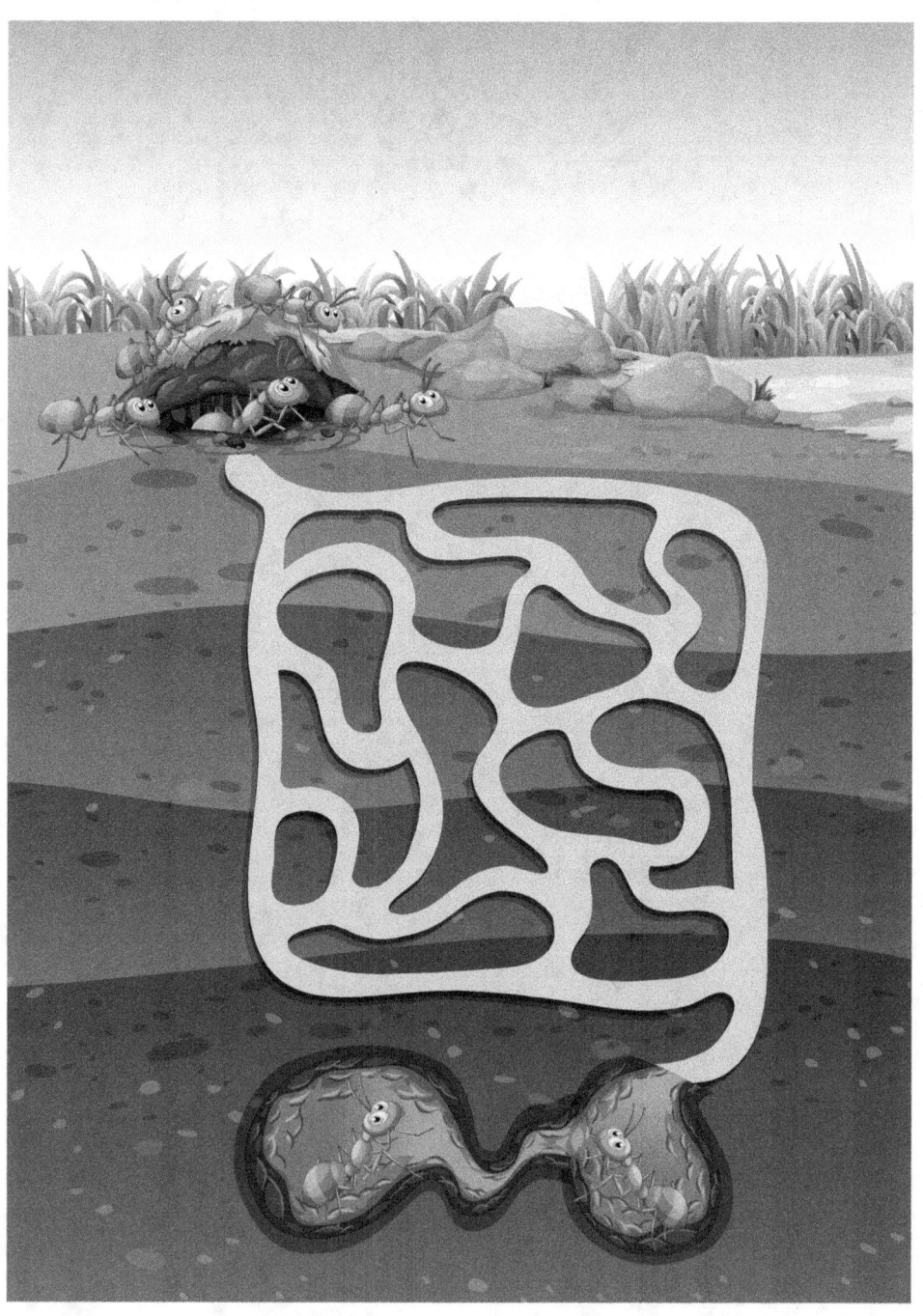

CAN YOU WRITE THE NAMES OF FRUITS?

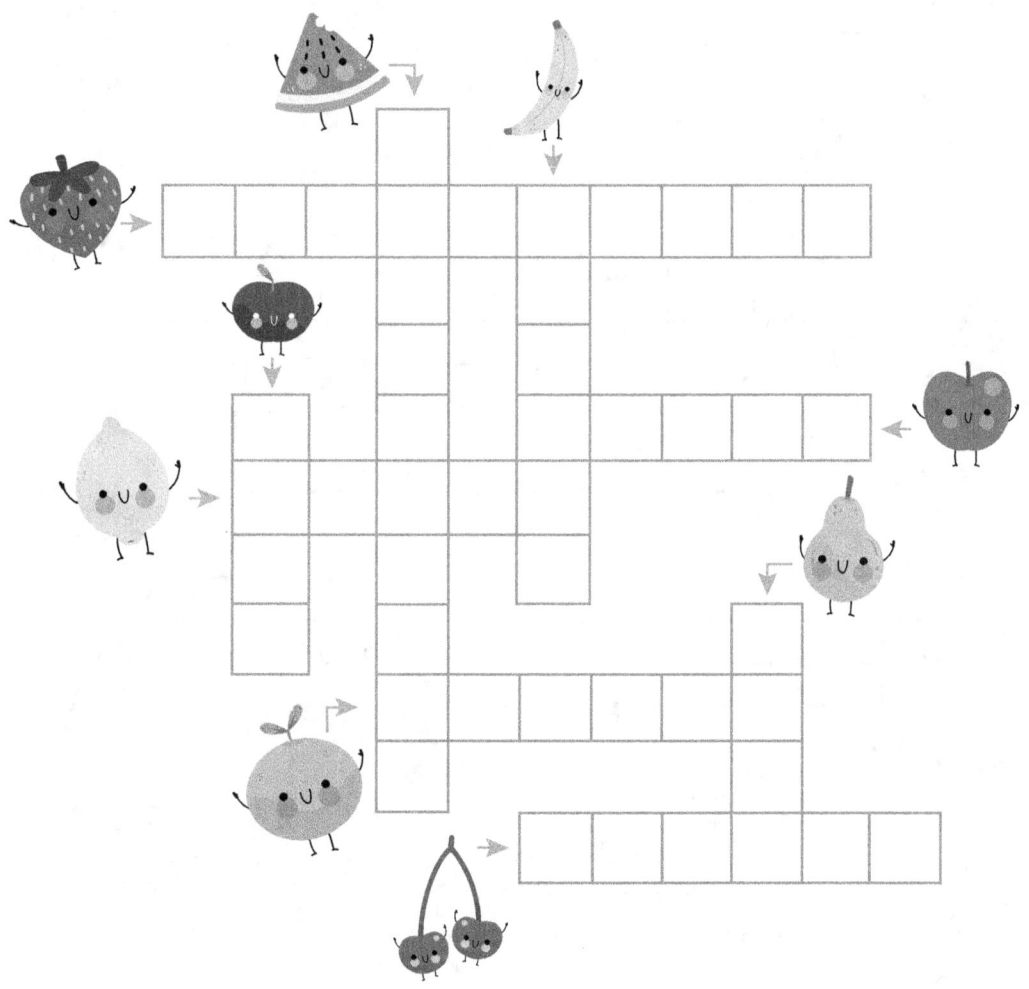

WRITE THE NAMES OF VARIOUS MODES OF TRANSPORT ACCORDING TO PICTURES.

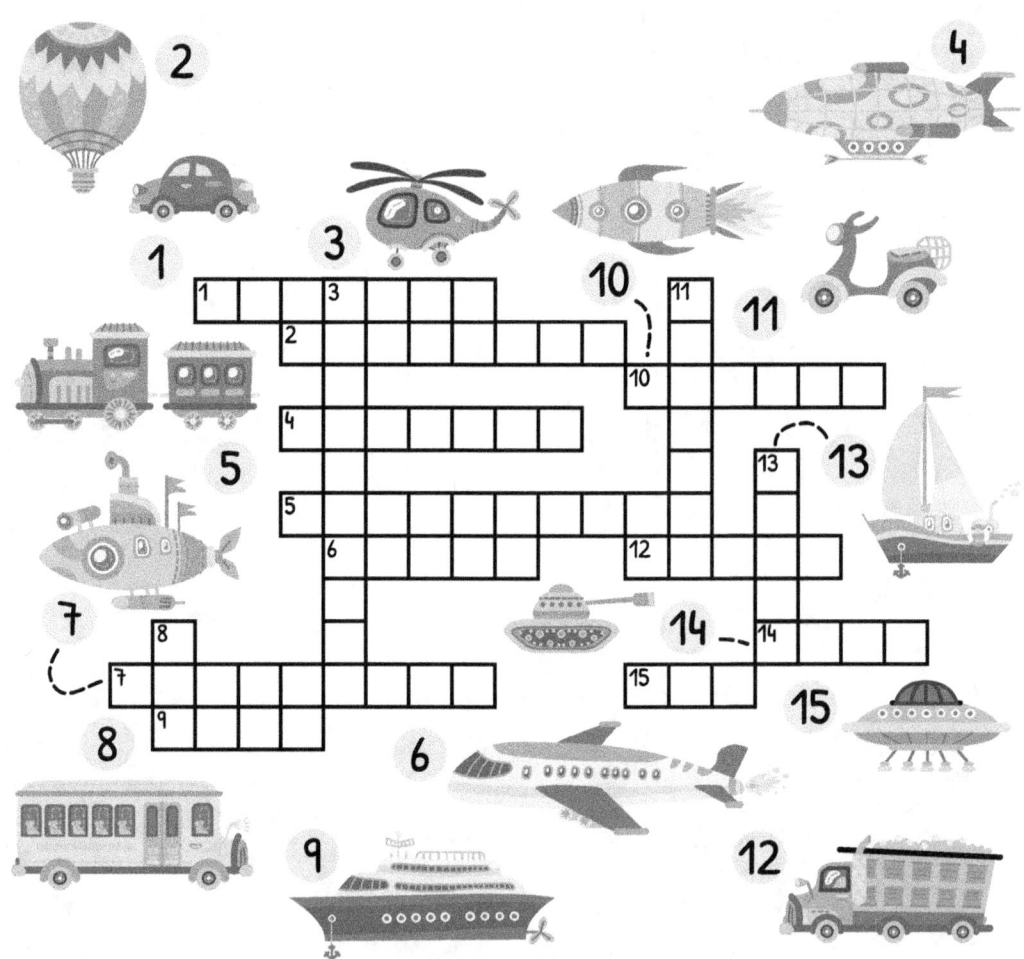

1.machine 2.aerostat 3.helicopter 4.airship 5.locomotive 6.plane 7.submarine 8.bus 9.ship 10.rocket 11.scooter 12.truck 13.yacht 14.tank 15.ufo

EVERY COLUMN, ROW, AND INNER UNIT (9 SQUARES) MUST BE WRITTEN WITH DIGITS 1 - 9 WITHOUT REPEATING ANY DIGITS.

	6	5	3	1		9		7
4					6	8		
	1		7	8		6		4
3		2		9	8			5
		8						
6		4	1	5			8	
5	2		8		7			9
		6	2	3			7	
	8		5		9		6	

EVERY COLUMN AND ROW HAS EMOJIS. FILL THE MISSING SPACES WITH SUITABLE EMOJIS.

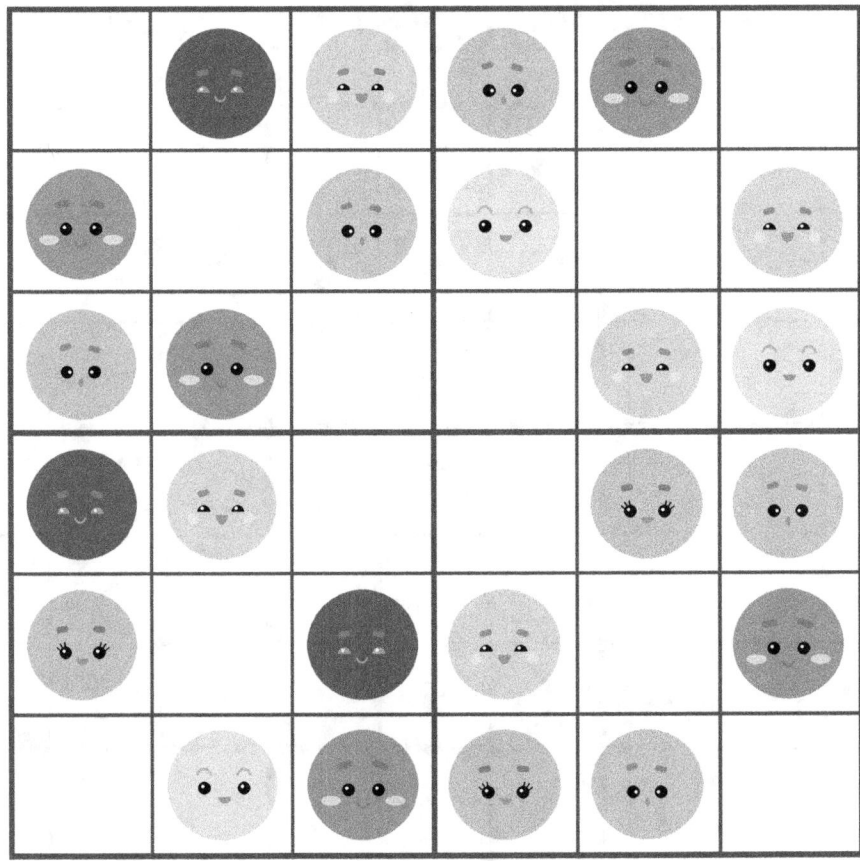

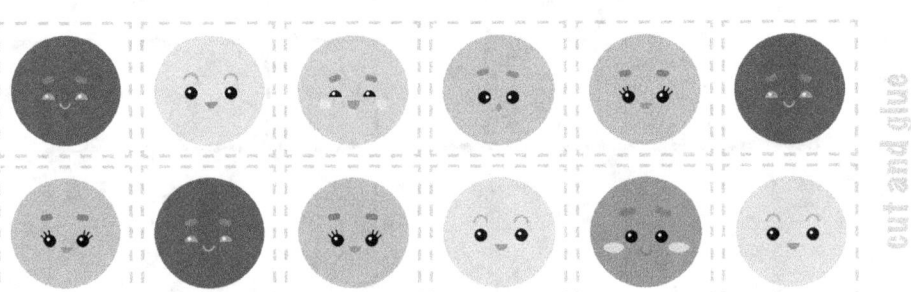

FIND THE ODD PUMPKIN

Can you find one Jack-o'-lantern different from the rest?

WHAT'S FOLLOWING?

There's a pattern to the pictures. Can you find out the series and select the right image that comes after from the pictures A, B, C, D, E, and F?

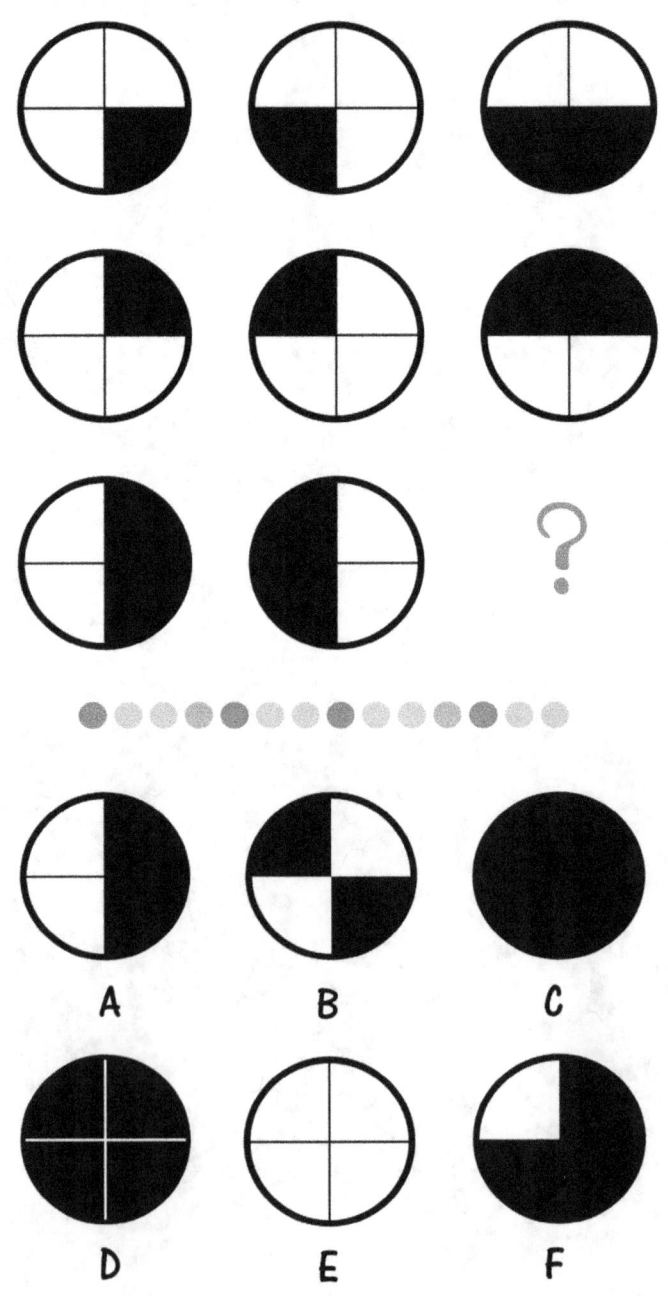

A   B   C

D   E   F

LOVE IS IN THE AIR

Find the following words about love. They may be hidden in all directions.

TREASURE   ATTRACTION

ADMIRE   BESOTTED

IDOLIZE   FLIRT

SWEETHEART   KISS

AFFECTION   ROMANCE

HEART   MARRIAGE

CHERISH   HUG

CRUSH

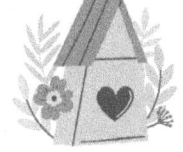

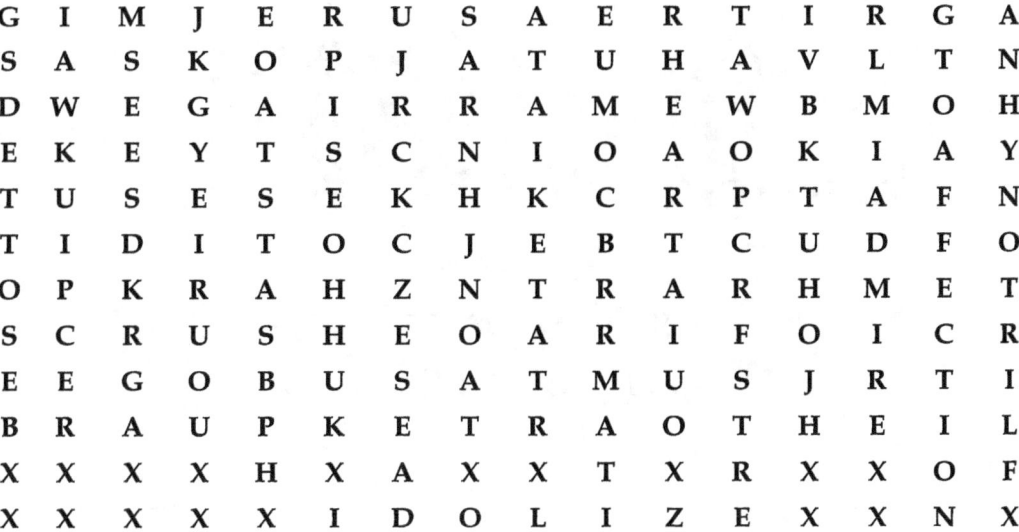

```
G  I  M  J  E  R  U  S  A  E  R  T  I  R  G  A
S  A  S  K  O  P  J  A  T  U  H  A  V  L  T  N
D  W  E  G  A  I  R  R  A  M  E  W  B  M  O  H
E  K  E  Y  T  S  C  N  I  O  A  O  K  I  A  Y
T  U  S  E  S  E  K  H  K  C  R  P  T  A  F  N
T  I  D  I  T  O  C  J  E  B  T  C  U  D  F  O
O  P  K  R  A  H  Z  N  T  R  A  R  H  M  E  T
S  C  R  U  S  H  E  O  A  R  I  F  O  I  C  R
E  E  G  O  B  U  S  A  T  M  U  S  J  R  T  I
B  R  A  U  P  K  E  T  R  A  O  T  H  E  I  L
X  X  X  X  H  X  A  X  X  T  X  R  X  X  O  F
X  X  X  X  X  I  D  O  L  I  Z  E  X  X  N  X
```

105

FIND THE INVENTION

Find the given words in the puzzle.

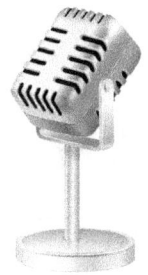

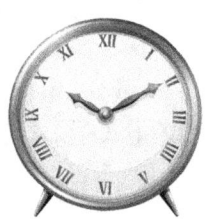

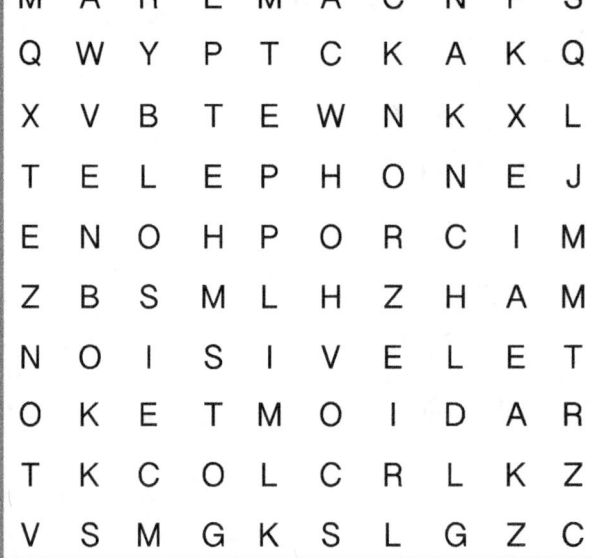

M	A	R	E	M	A	C	N	F	S
Q	W	Y	P	T	C	K	A	K	Q
X	V	B	T	E	W	N	K	X	L
T	E	L	E	P	H	O	N	E	J
E	N	O	H	P	O	R	C	I	M
Z	B	S	M	L	H	Z	H	A	M
N	O	I	S	I	V	E	L	E	T
O	K	E	T	M	O	I	D	A	R
T	K	C	O	L	C	R	L	K	Z
V	S	M	G	K	S	L	G	Z	C

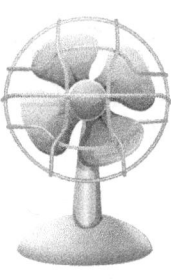

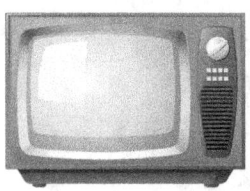

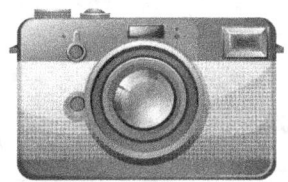

**CAMERA - MICROPHONE - TELEVISION -
TELEPHONE - CLOCK - FAN**

PART - IV
4. Memory Activities for Seniors Coping with Dementia

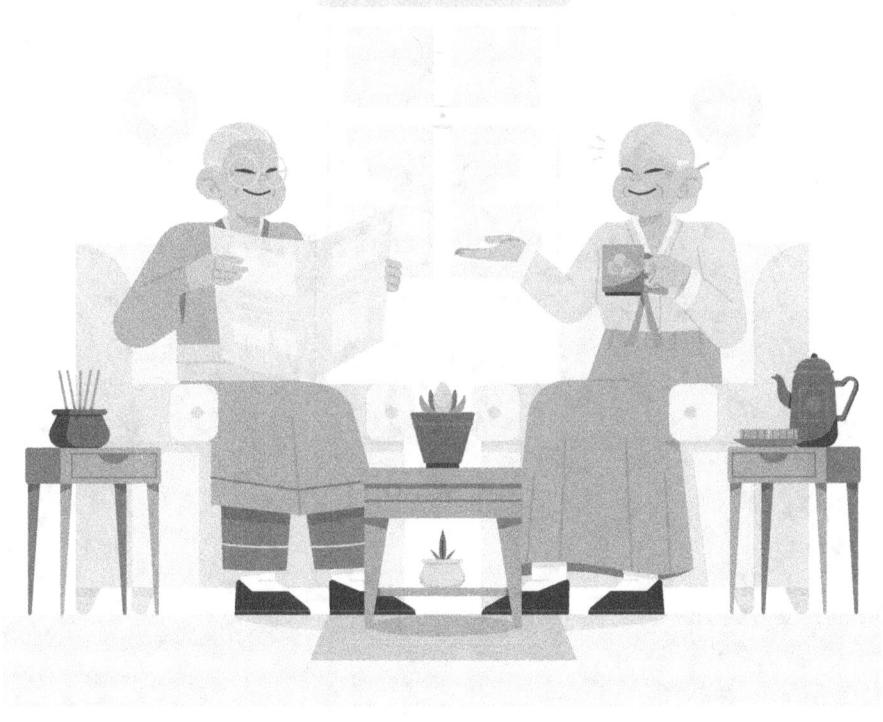

Due to dementia, you are more likely to lose the capacity to remember words and names other than your childhood memories. Most of you with dementia can recall your school time or wedding day. That's why memory exercises have the potential to develop positive sentiments by tapping into long-term happy memories.

Memory activities can comprise life experiences and tales from the past. Sharing such stories with your dear ones can also bring a purpose of value and help you reconnect with positive memories. Allow your listeners to ask questions instead of getting confused or frustrated.

The following poster is specially designed to show you activities that can help to enhance your memory; you can make them a daily part of your routine.

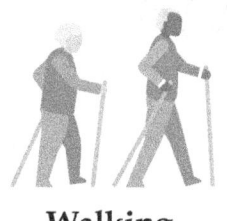

Walking

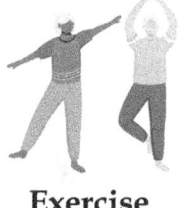

Exercise

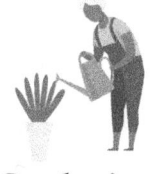

Gardening

Activities for Improving Memory

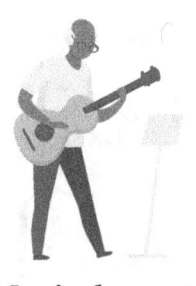

Book Reading

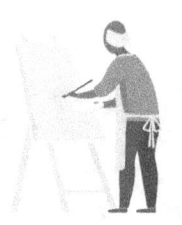

Art and crafts

Musical events

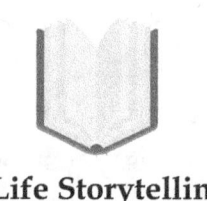

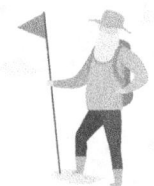

Physical exercise and sports

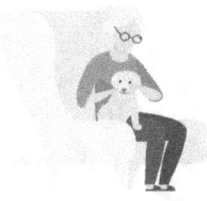

Life Storytelling

Pet Therapy

4.1. Mealtime Routines

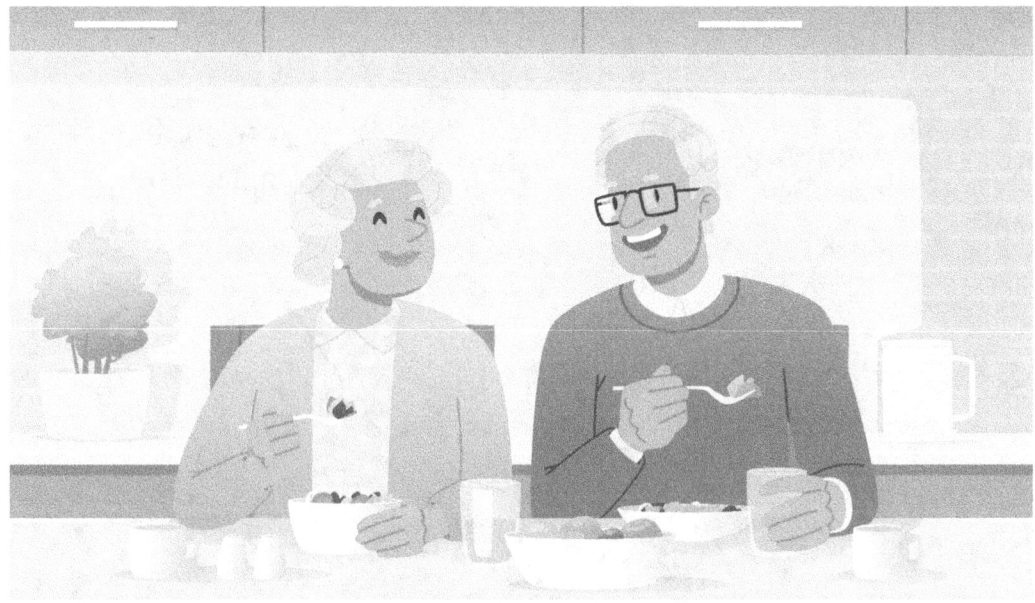

Scheduled mealtimes are a fantastic practice. The routine creates procedural memory with your community members; you can organize an event outside or a regularly scheduled teatime.

Consider incorporating each of the senses into mealtimes when scheduling mealtime routine activities. Food is more than taste! Focus on the pleasant aroma of the meat you are roasting for the event, the sizzling sound of cutlets frying, or the incredible smoothness of pizza dough being kneaded. Try to set the plate deliciously to your eyes, and try to recall and share your memories.

The following picture depicts what is healthy eating for you. Look at it carefully and try to incorporate these items into your daily meal.

Do not skip
breakfast

Eat fruits and
veggies daily

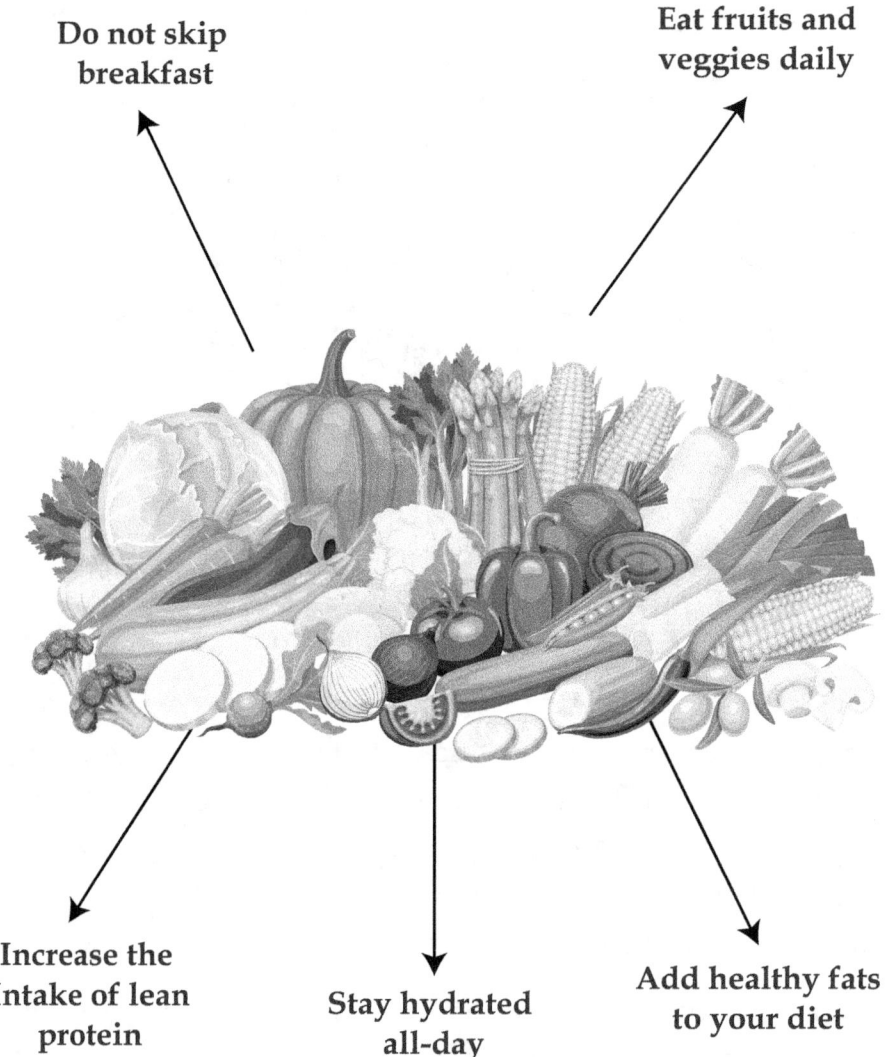

Increase the
Intake of lean
protein

Stay hydrated
all-day

Add healthy fats
to your diet

Before going further, let's make a meal plan for a week; while planning, ensure you include all the essential nutrients for a healthy diet.

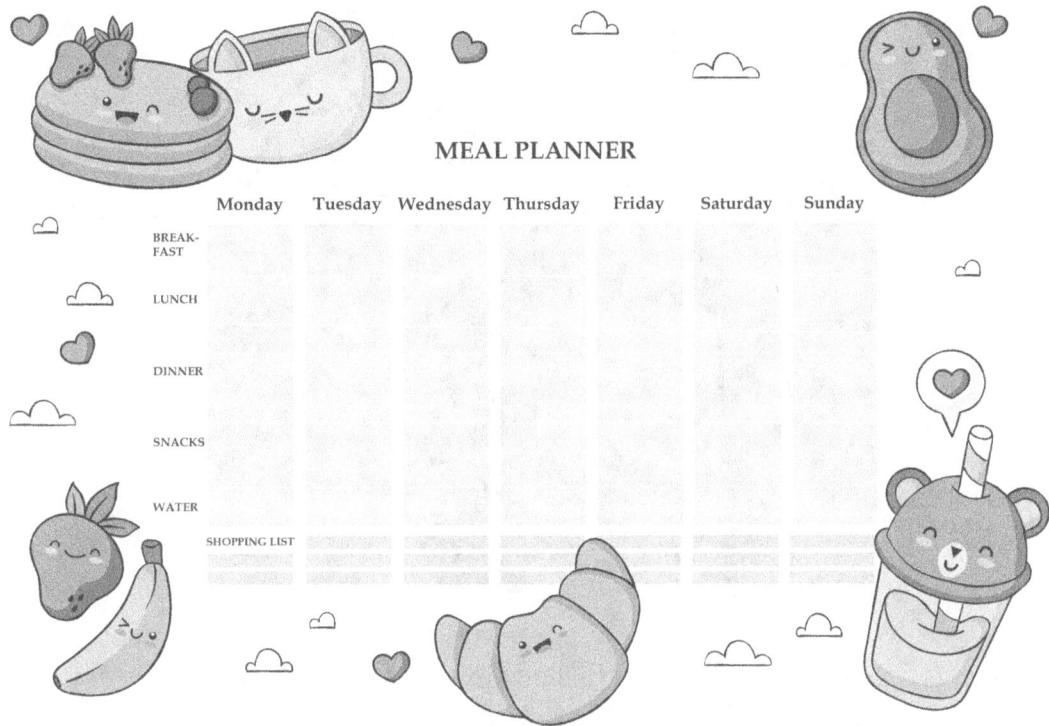

MEAL PLANNER

	Monday	Tuesday	Wednesday	Thursday	Friday	Saturday	Sunday
BREAK-FAST							
LUNCH							
DINNER							
SNACKS							
WATER							

SHOPPING LIST

4.2. Singing/Music

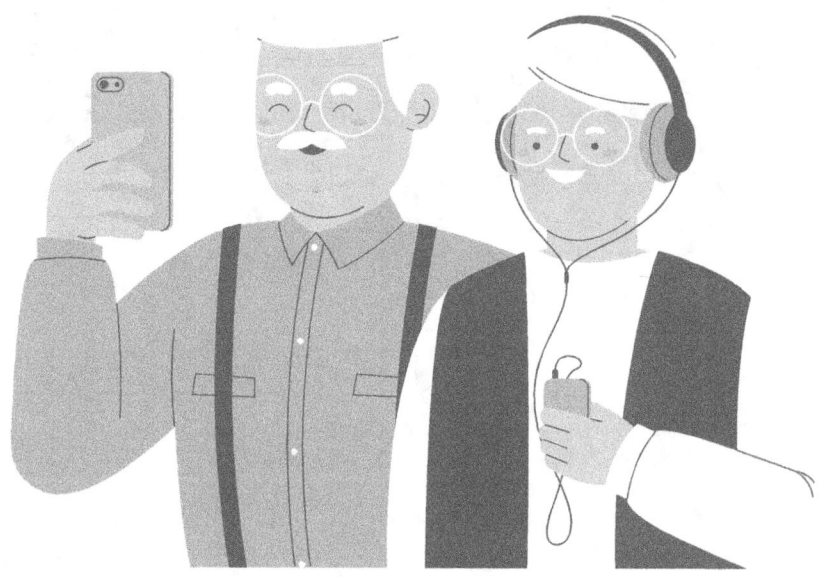

Music is a fantastic therapy; it has a calming and pacifying effect. Music unleashes dopamine, a chemical produced in the brain, which is linked with enjoyment and pleasure. Investigations have revealed that dementia patients showed a substantial decrease in tension after 6 weeks of music therapy.

Other investigations have uncovered that music therapy can help you with dementia, remember memories and provide moments of clarity. For those who have appreciated music, listening to classics or singing unforgettable songs and vacation carols may return memories of earlier days. Music programs and music-related activities are excellent for you. Following are six music-based activities for you that will support your health, joy, and longevity.

1. **Karaoke**
2. **Dance**
3. **Musical Chairs**
4. **Guess That Song**
5. **Drum Circle**
6. **Musical Storytelling**

Find the way.

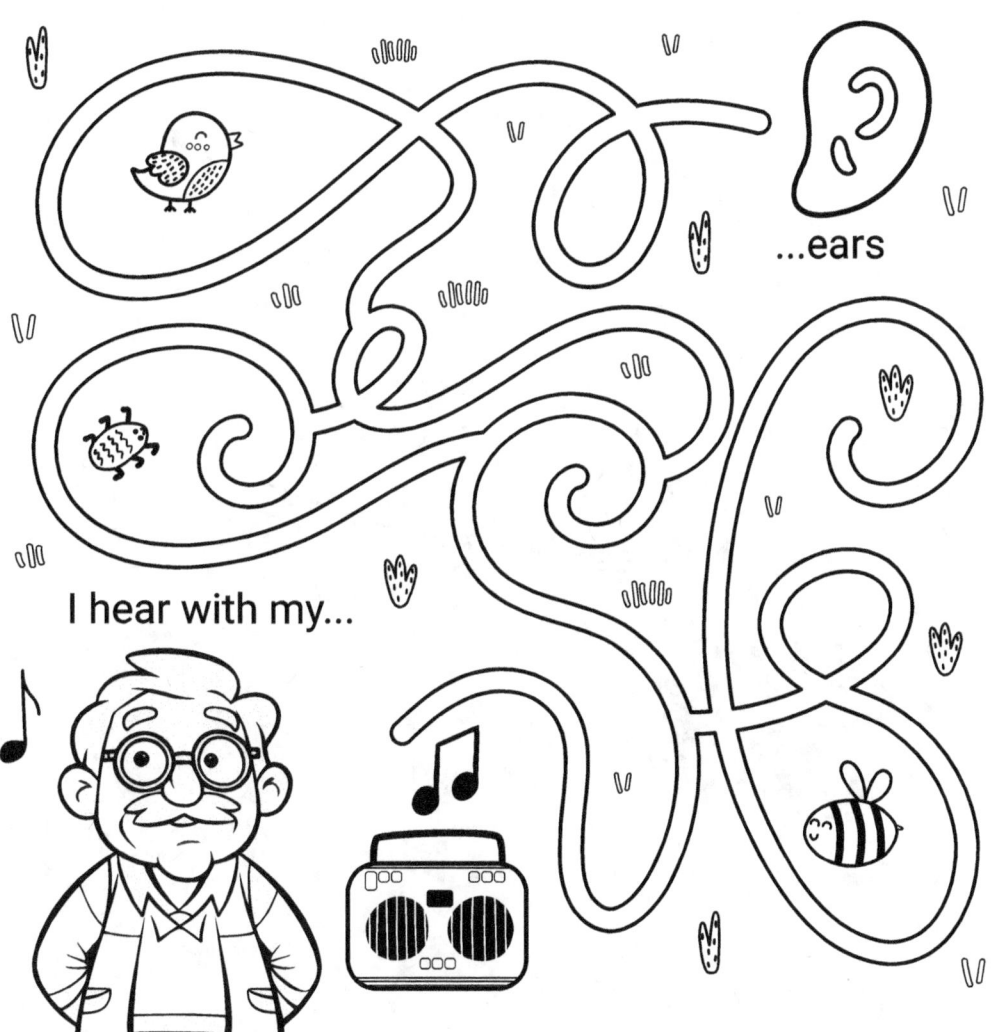

...ears

I hear with my...

CAN YOU TRACE THE LINES AND COLOR THE DRUM?

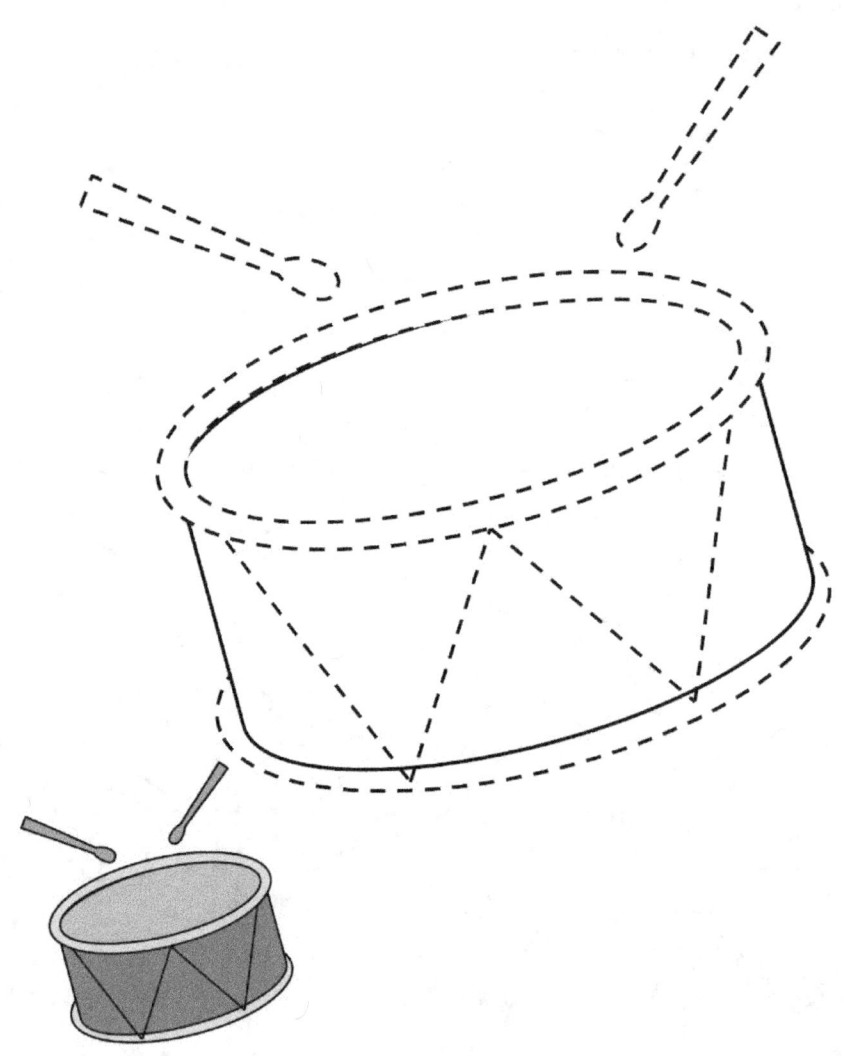

4.3. Historic Activities

These activities are a combination of multiple sensory items set to stimulate memories revolving around your past, like:

- ✓ Making a memory box
- ✓ Watching classic movies
- ✓ Going through or creating picture albums and
- ✓ Glancing at old magazines or catalogs

It can be an excellent way to recall your life history, interests and values. My dear seniors, there must be organized programs in your community by the authorities to help you stay active and fit. Senior Services of America is devoted to supplying the best personal care and activities for all seniors with dementia.

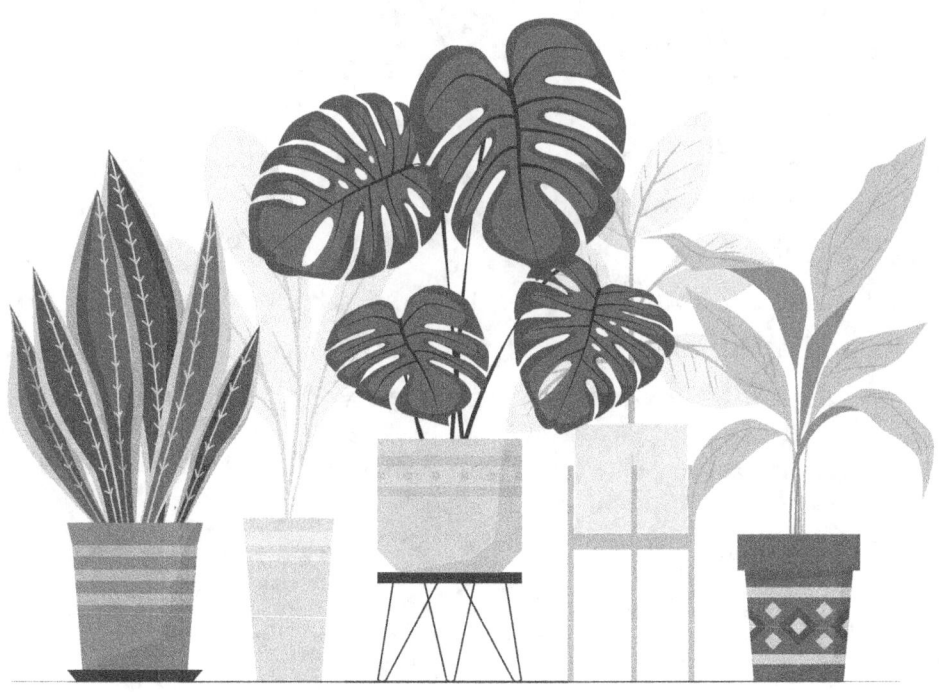

4.4. Mindfulness Break

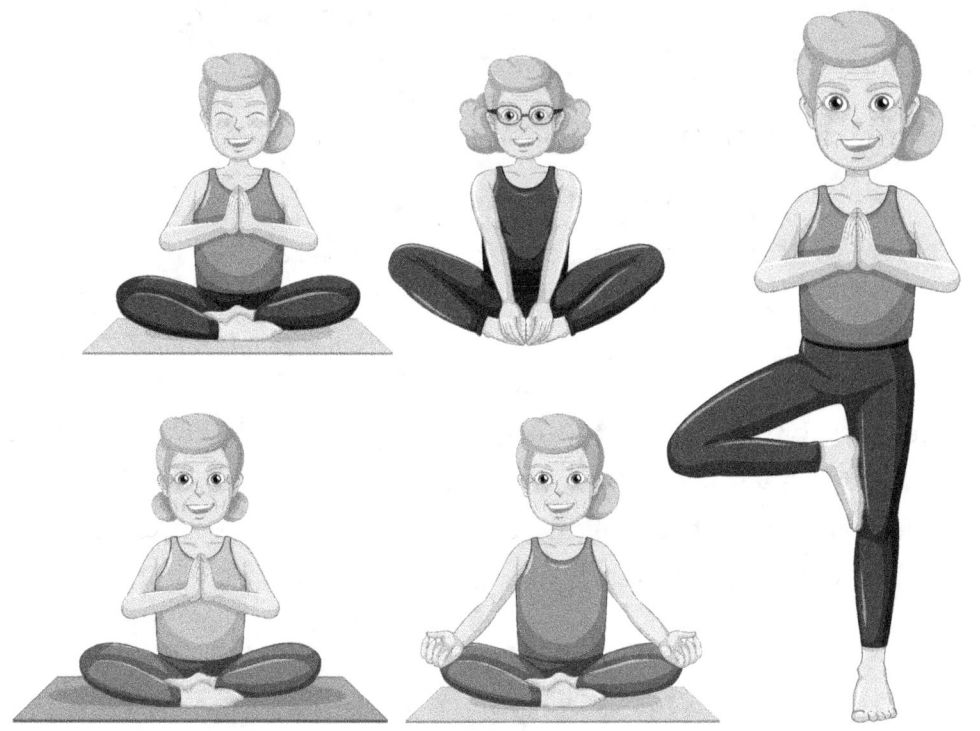

Yoga and meditation have a long and interconnected history. When practicing yoga, you witness the sensations of your body as it progresses through freedom while having various positions and stretches. Concentrating on body movements is simultaneously a mindfulness exercise and a workout! Some of you initially feel threatened by yoga, but there are multiple variations, like chair yoga, that can be tailored to fulfill the needs of people at all levels of mobility.

Some famous chair yoga postures are mentioned in the following posters. You can also practice them, but before starting, consult your physician.

SENIOR CHAIR YOGA POSTURES

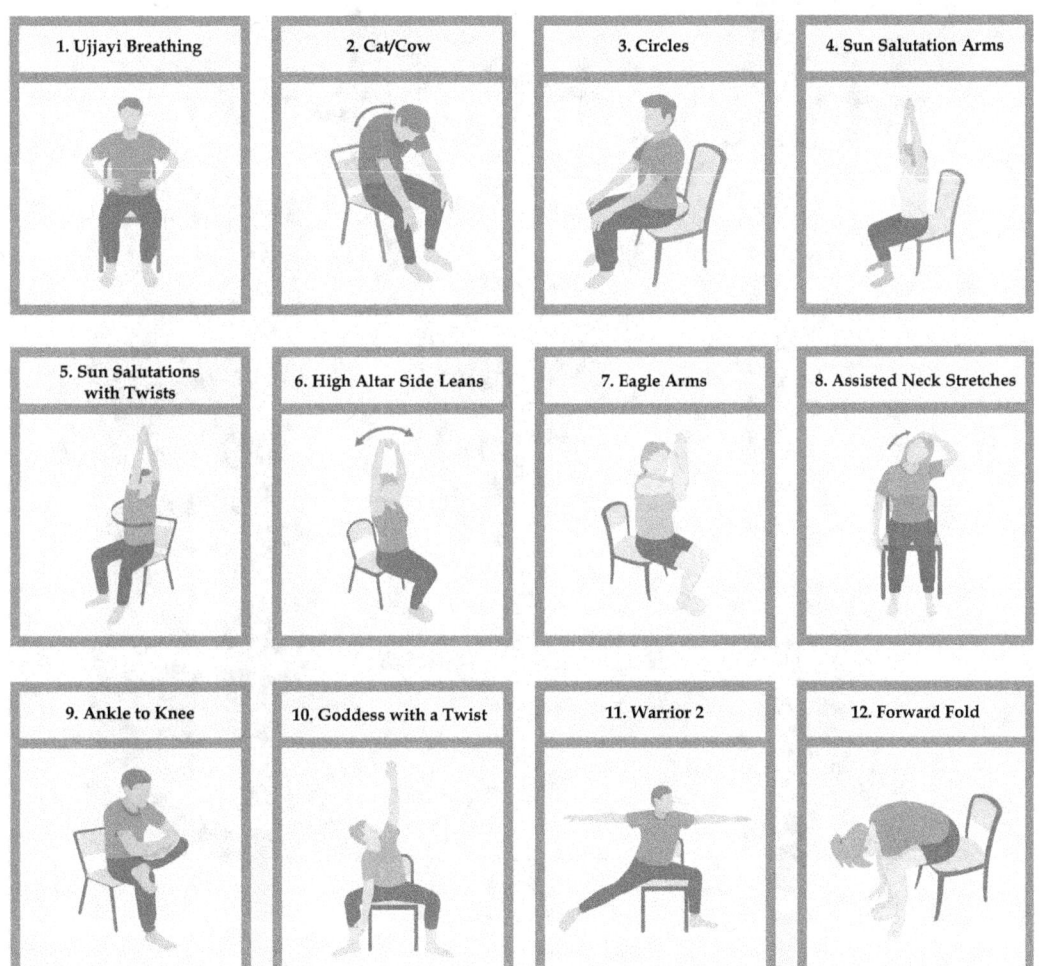

Bonus Brain Games

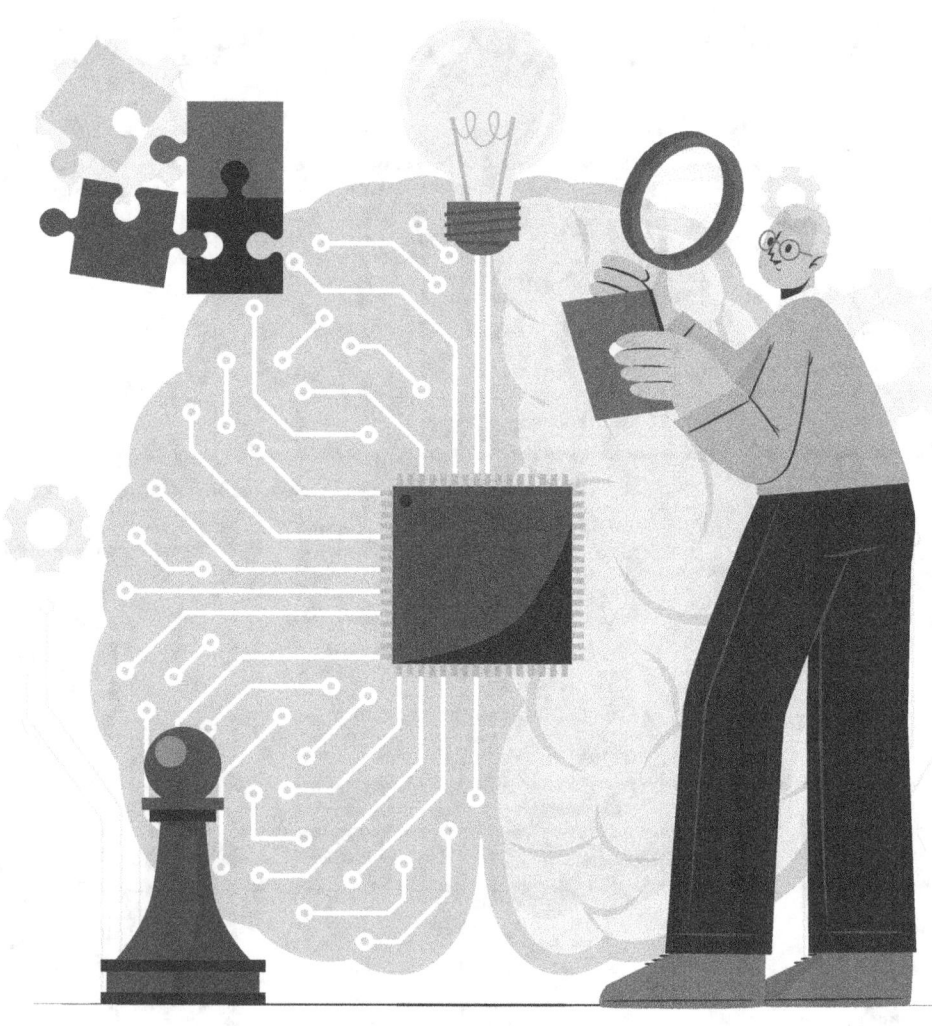

SHADOW MATCHING

Can you match the shadow with the picture?

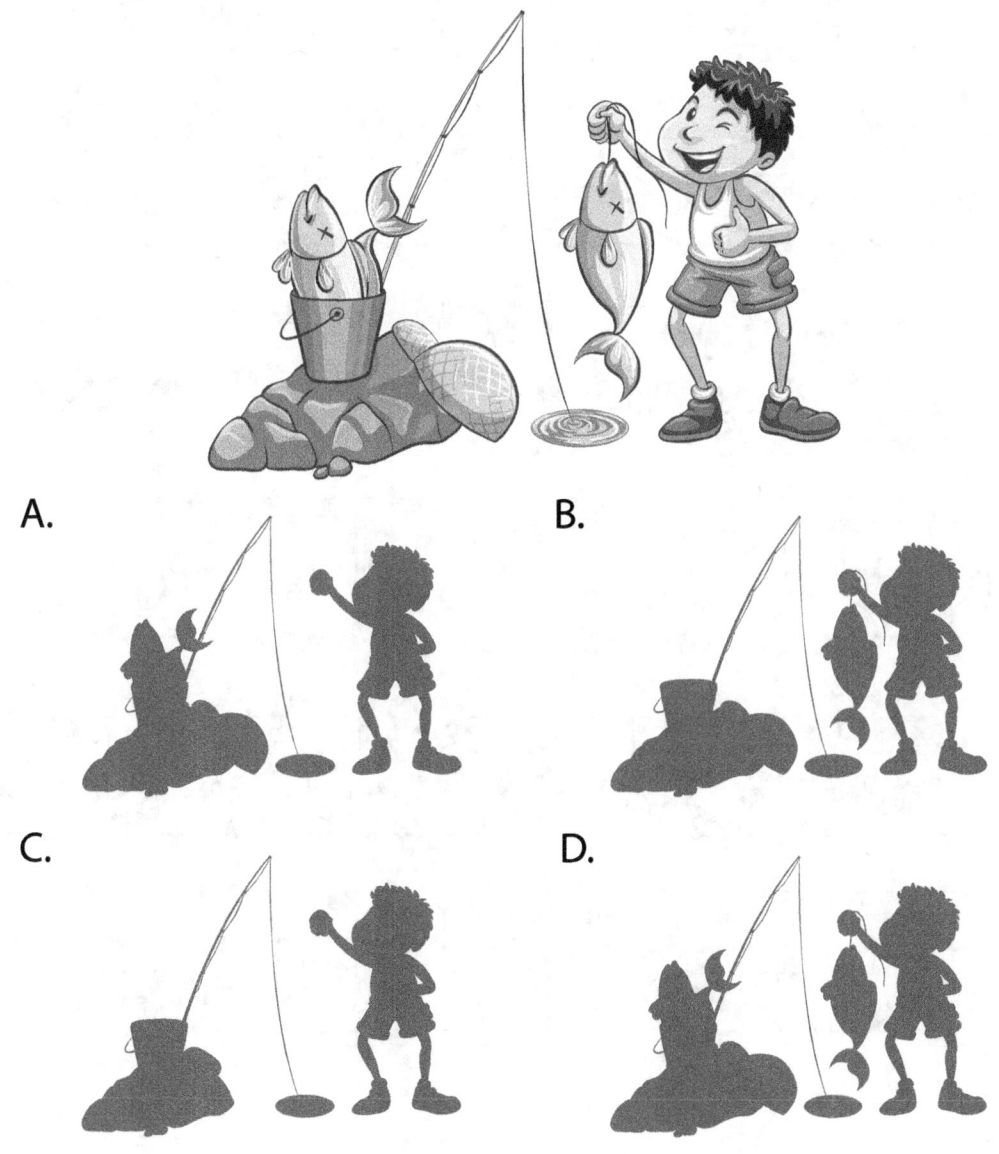

A.

B.

C.

D.

MATCHING TRAINS

Can you find the two identical trains?

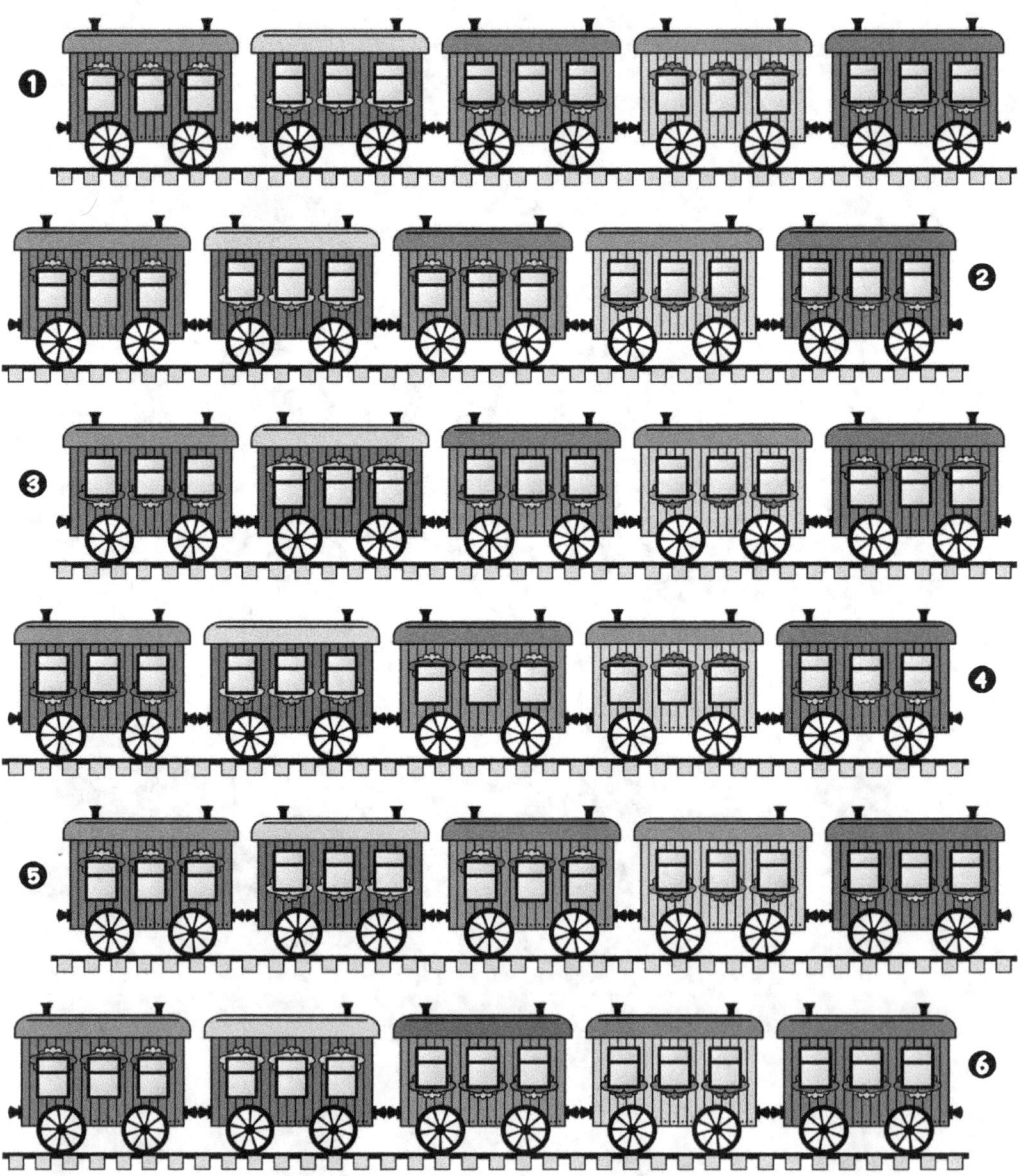

THE PERFECT KEY

Which one is the perfect key for the clock?

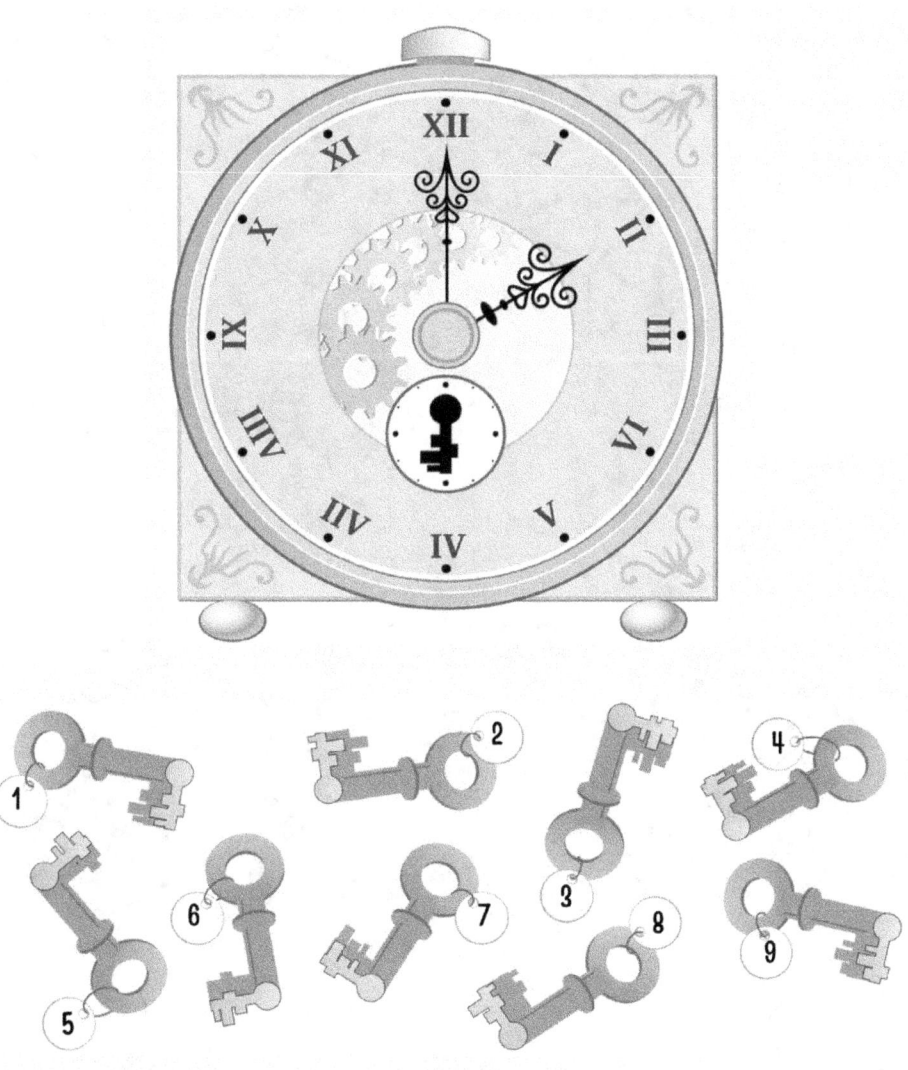

COMPLETE THE PUZZLE

Can you guess which 2 sections can be used to make picture no 3?

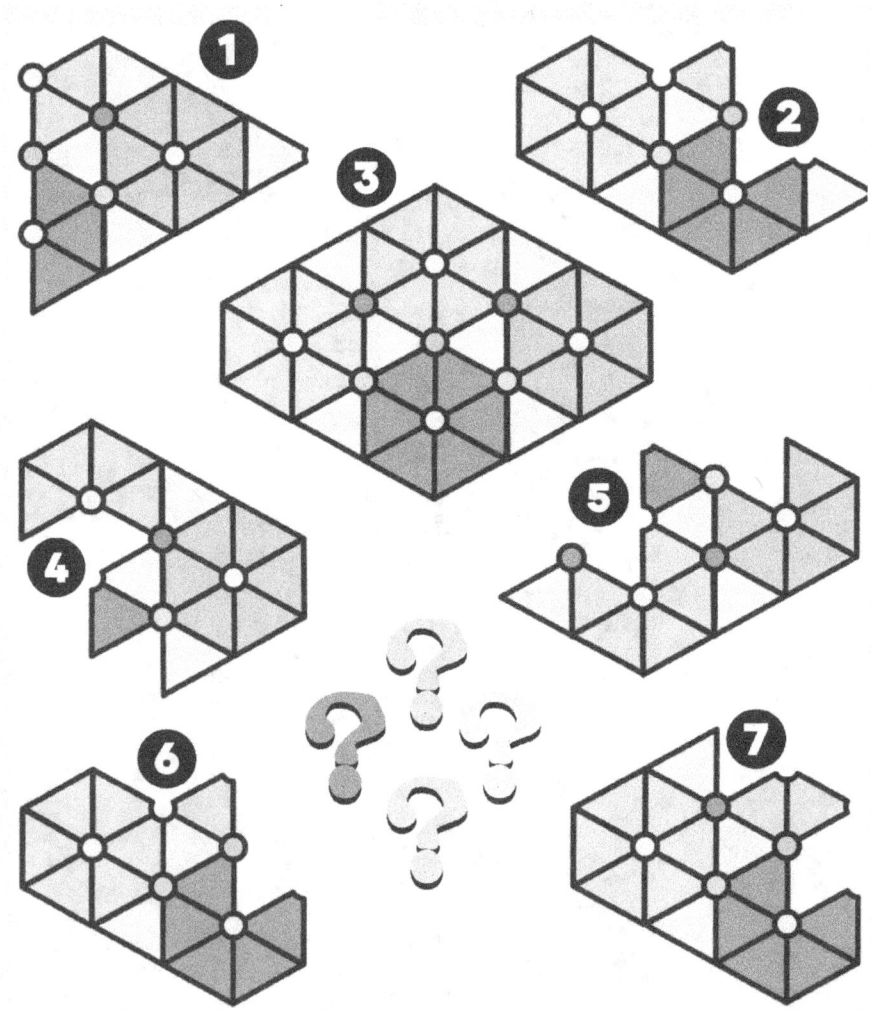

UNTANGLING THE NECKLACES

Which one of the four clasps must be opened to untangle all the necklaces?

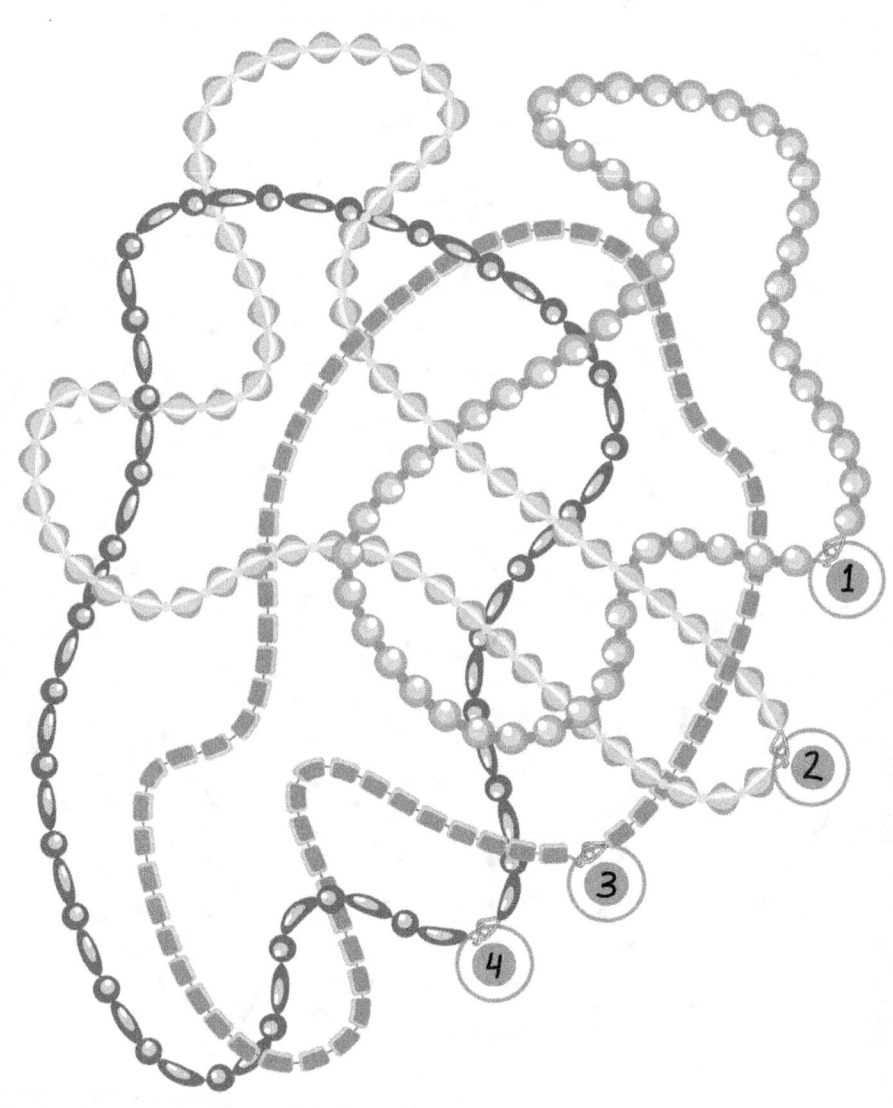

GRAB THE CHERRY!

Get the cherry to decorate your favorite dessert.

START

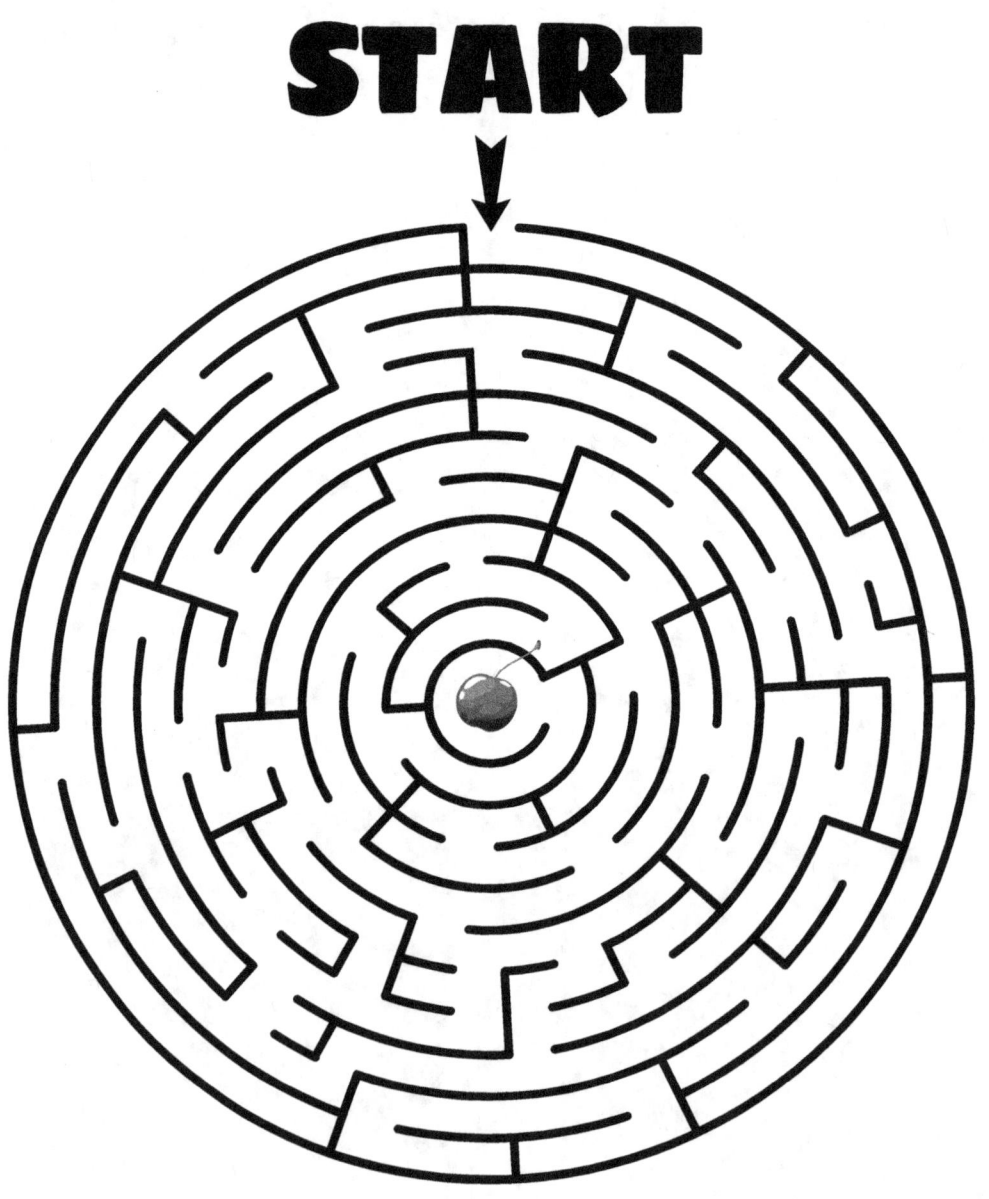

CAN YOU WRITE THE NAMES OF THE SPORTS?

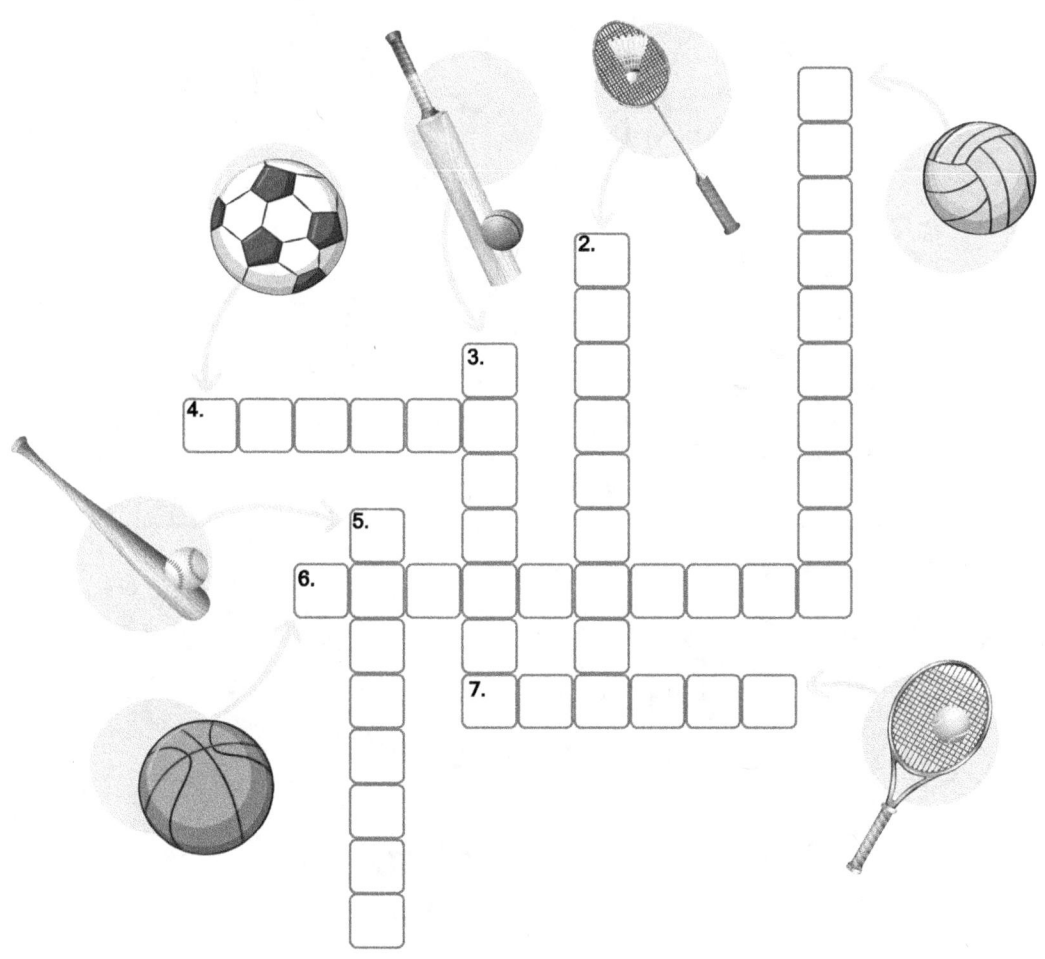

THE COLOR GAME

Complete the names of the colors.

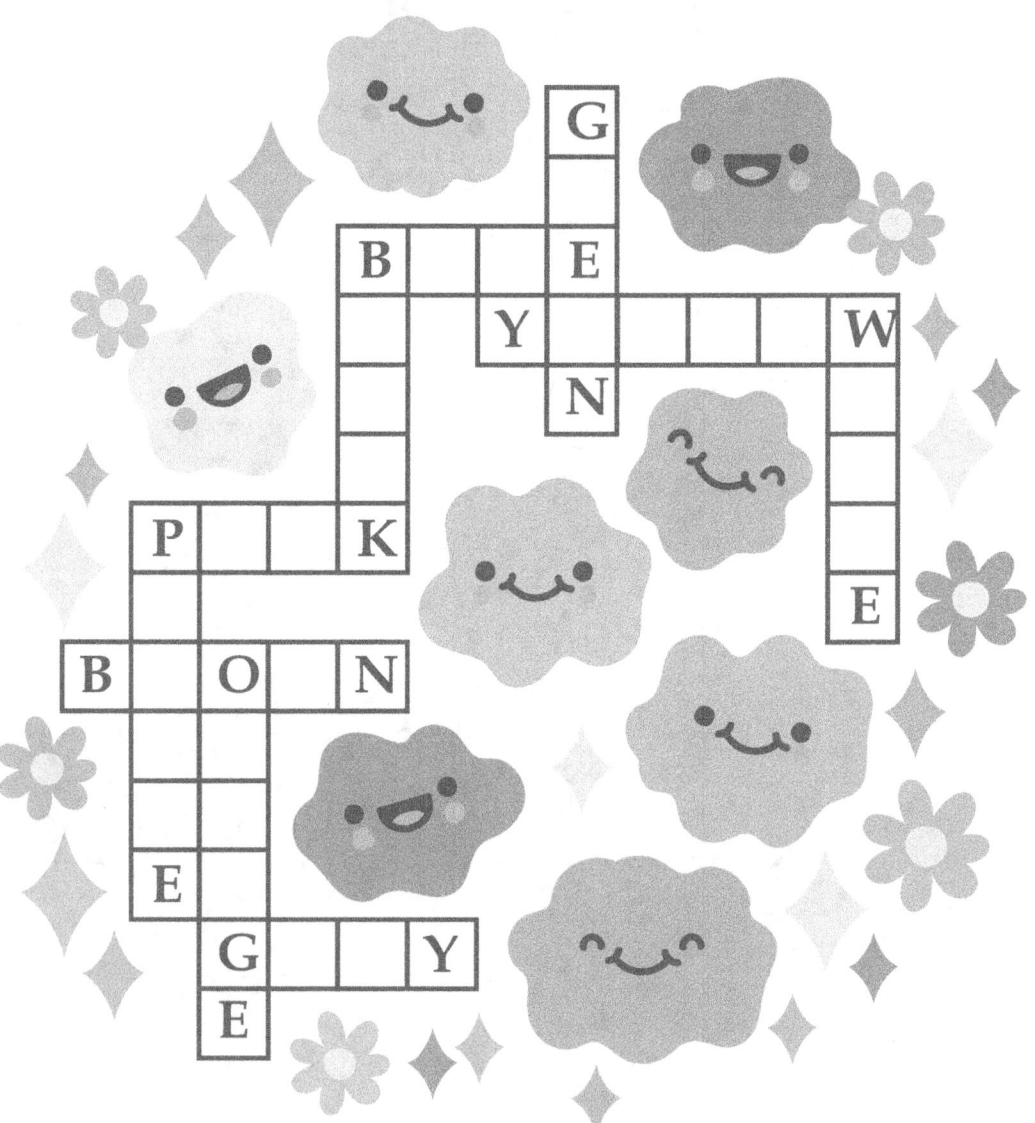

THE UMBRELLA MANIA

Find the correct top view of the colorful umbrella.

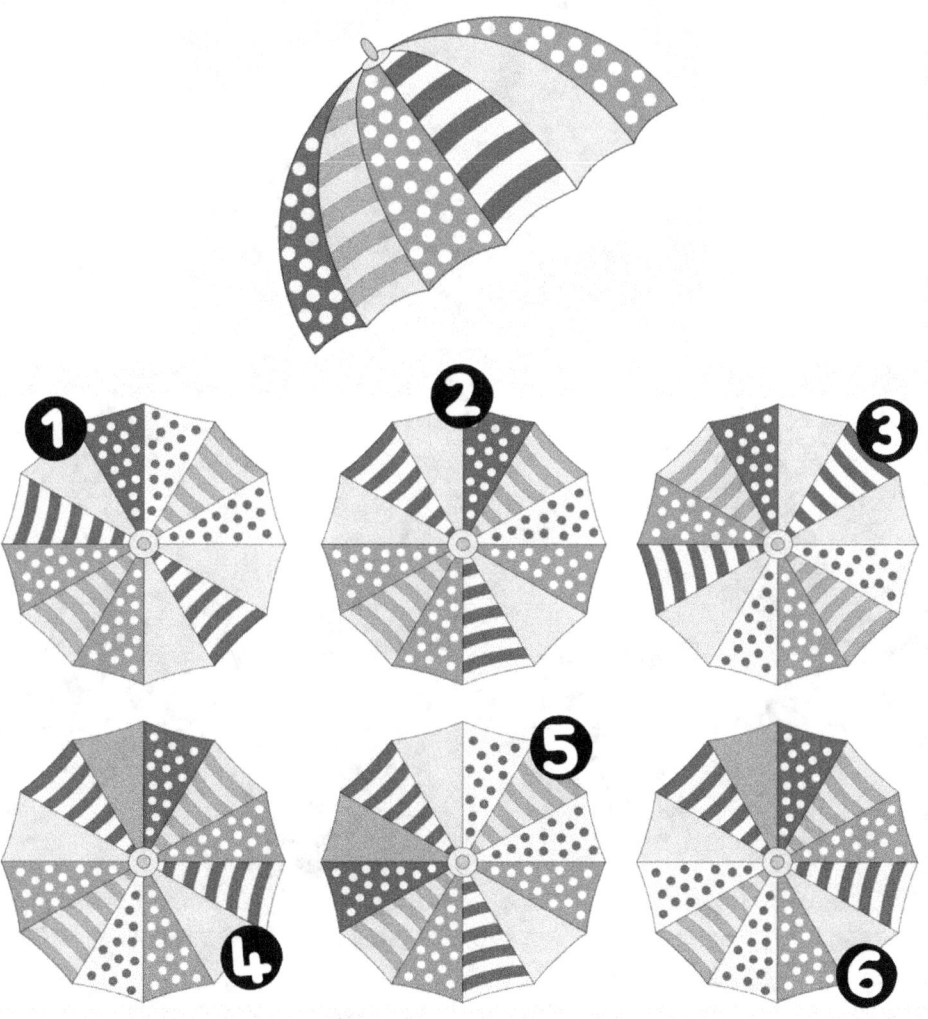

CHOOSE THE TOP SECTION FROM 1-8
TO COMPLETE THE PYRAMID.

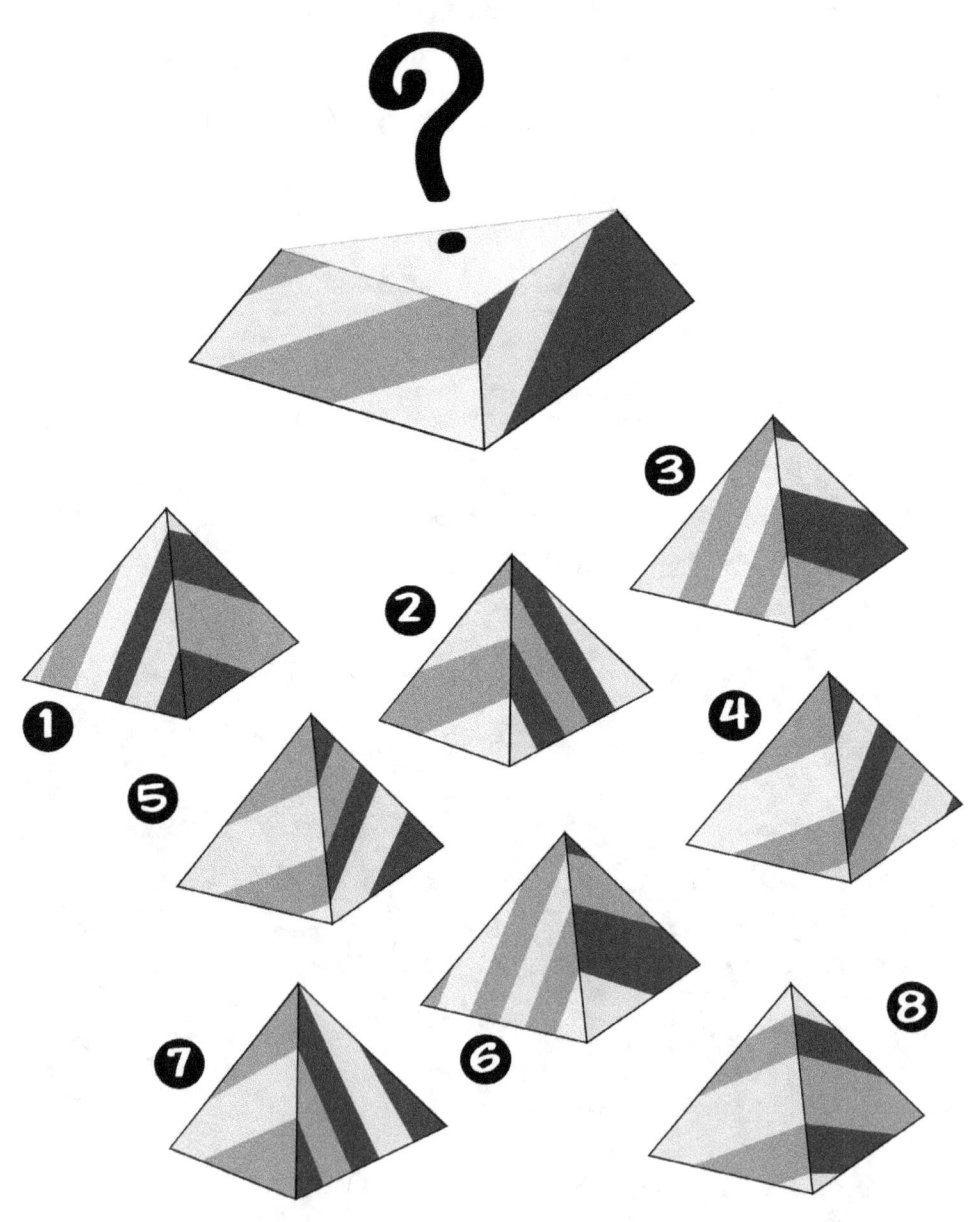

Draw lines around sections that contain 4 squares and 2 red circles by utilizing all the squares and circles.

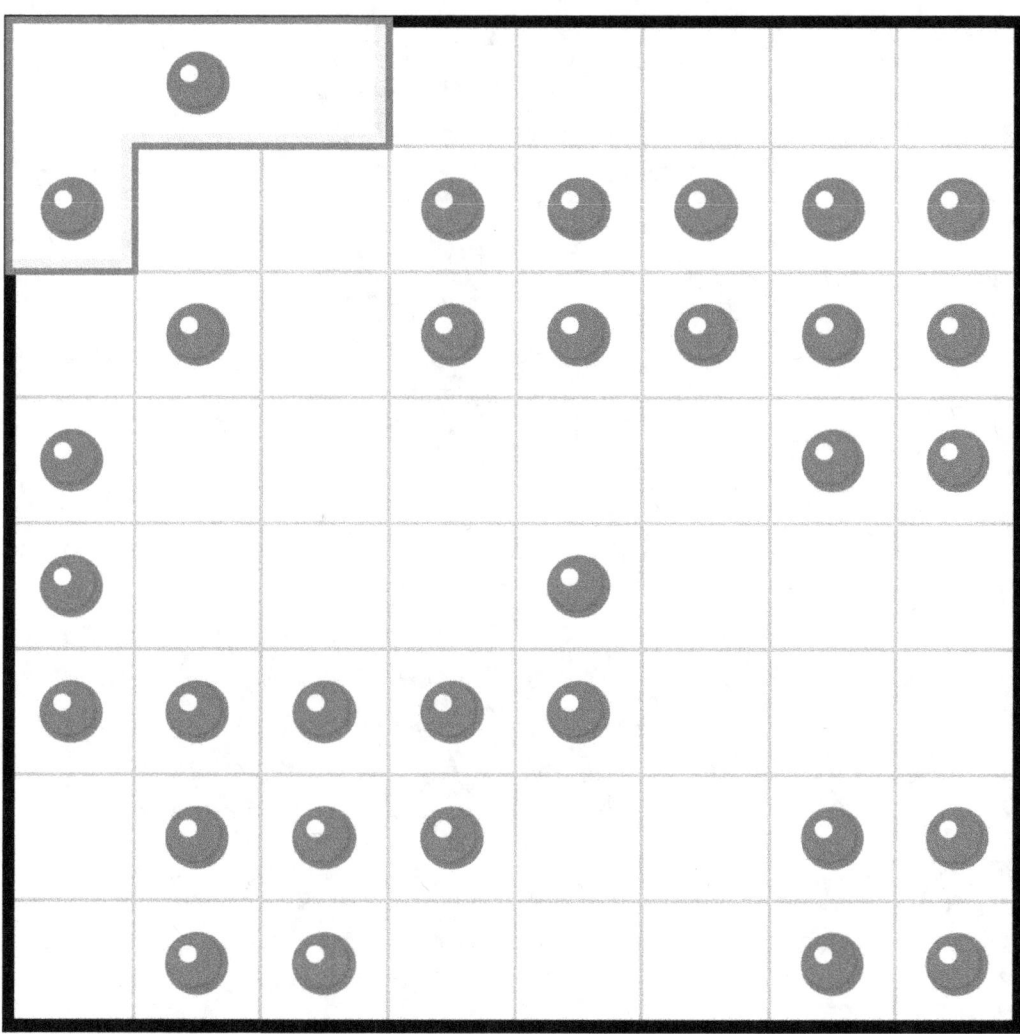

129

MAKE THE BOX

Can you find the five accurate sides that will join together to form the wooden box?

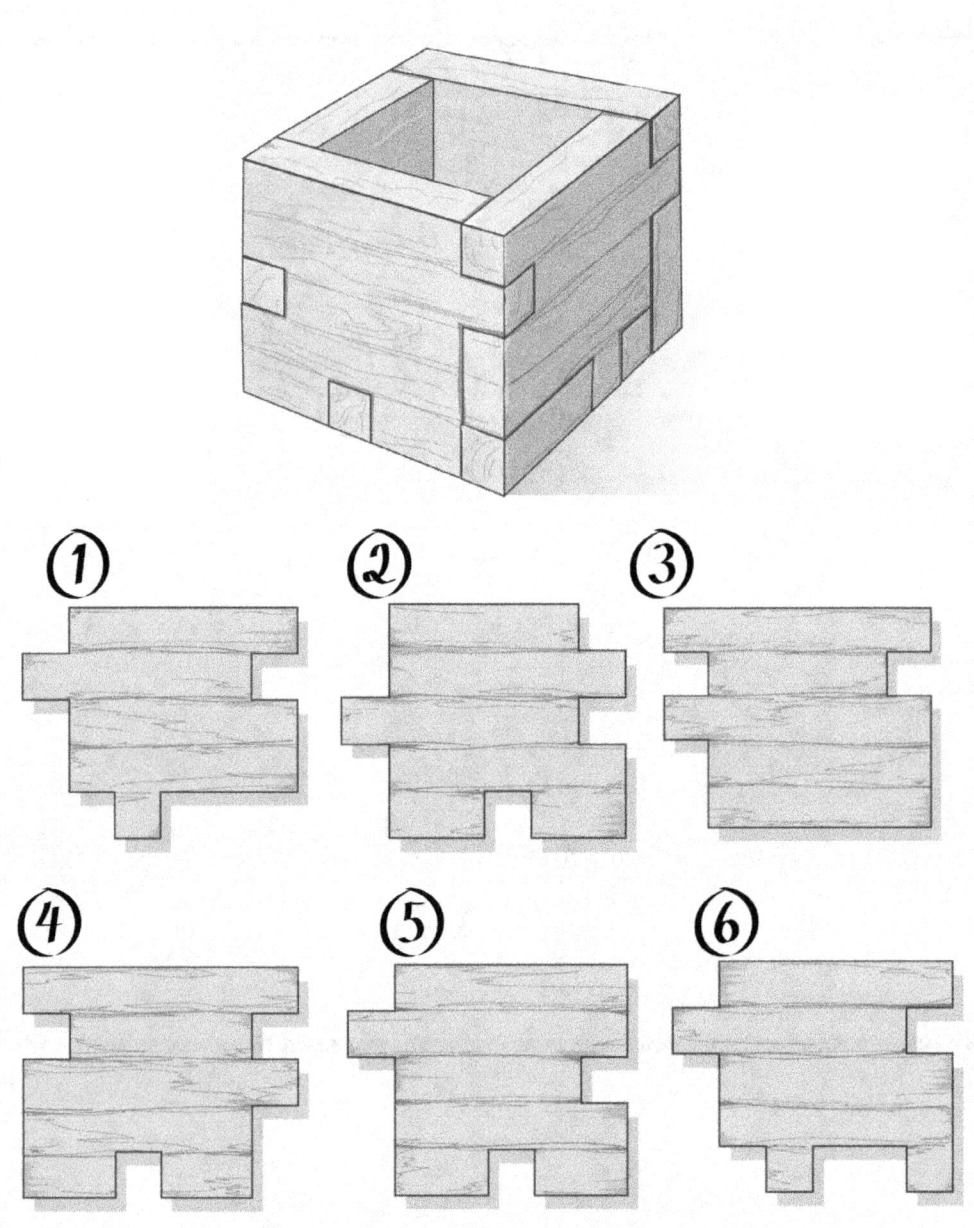

COUNTING THE WHEELS

Count the similar vehicles and write the total number of each vehicle.

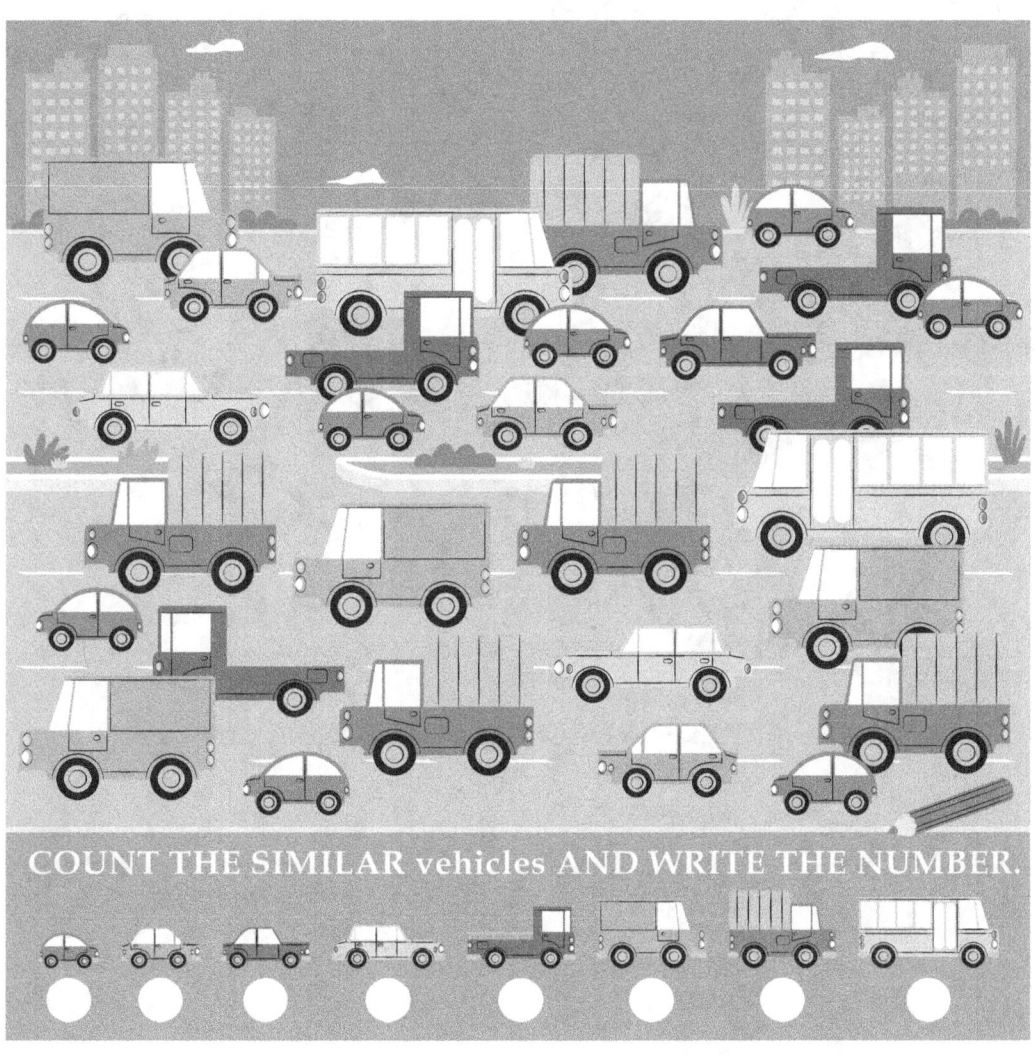

THE DINO COUNT

Count the similar dinosaurs and write the total number for each type.

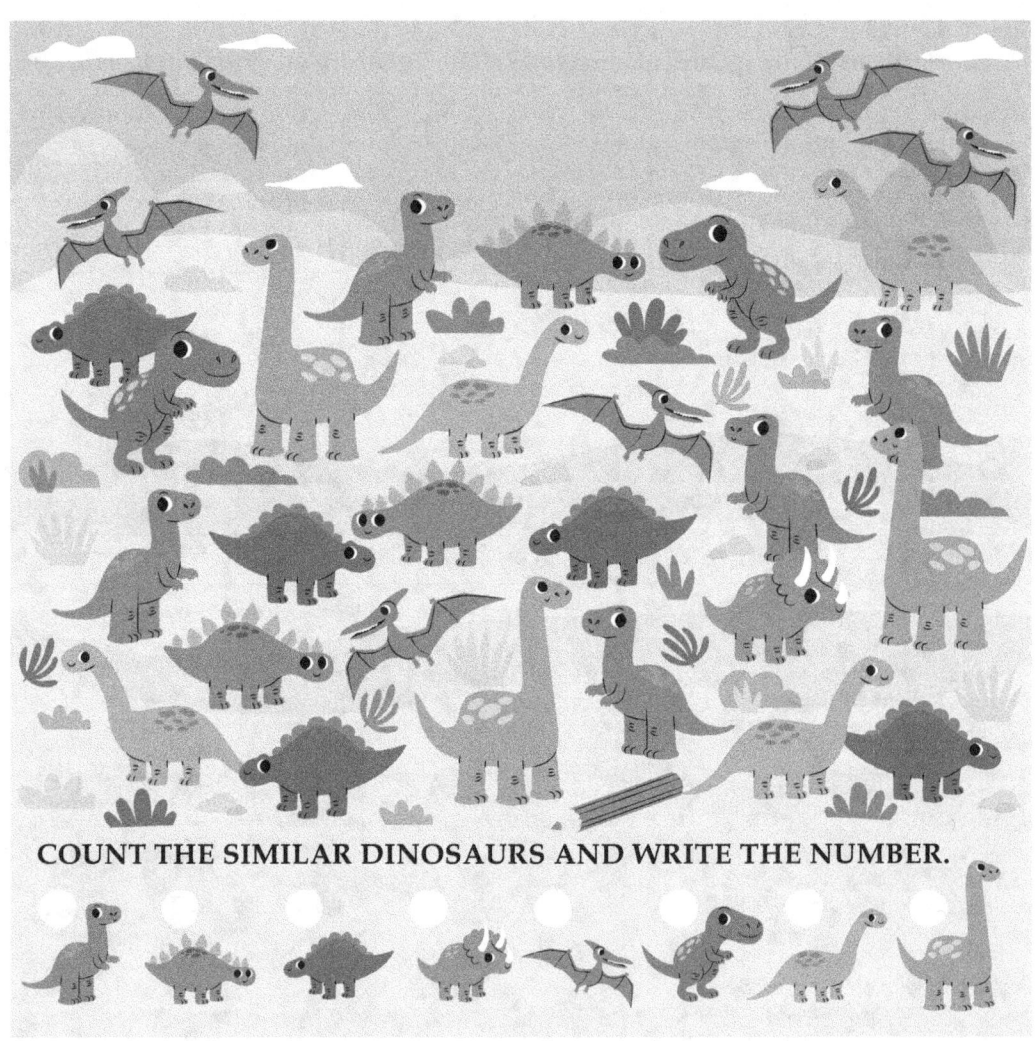

COUNT THE SIMILAR DINOSAURS AND WRITE THE NUMBER.

Reflecting on Progress

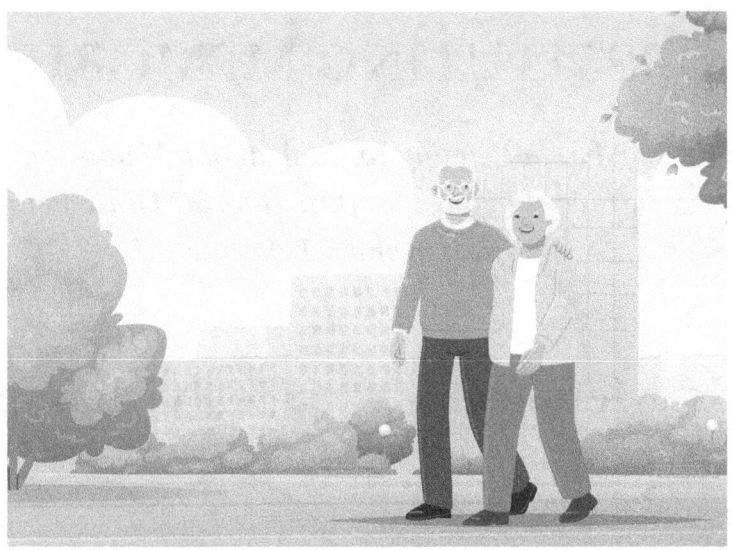

After performing all the above activities, one question arises: How do we judge our progress? You can achieve various benefits from successfully performing all the exercises, including improved mental health, fitness, strength and concentration. You can talk to your close friends or family about the positive changes you observe in yourself. Following are some indications that you have improved:

- ✓ Sweetened mood
- ✓ Sounder sleep
- ✓ Decreased constipation
- ✓ Improved motor skills
- ✓ Lowered risk of falls due to improved stability and strength
- ✓ Decreased decline rate in mental health
- ✓ Enhanced memory
- ✓ Improved behavior, such as a lowered rate of wandering and aggressiveness
- ✓ Sound communication and social skills

Reflection Time

SUBSTITUTING MEMORIES

Few memories can be challenging to think about. If you could re-design a memory, what would you substitute it with? Draw your old and fresh memory below.

Old Memory   **Fresh Memory**

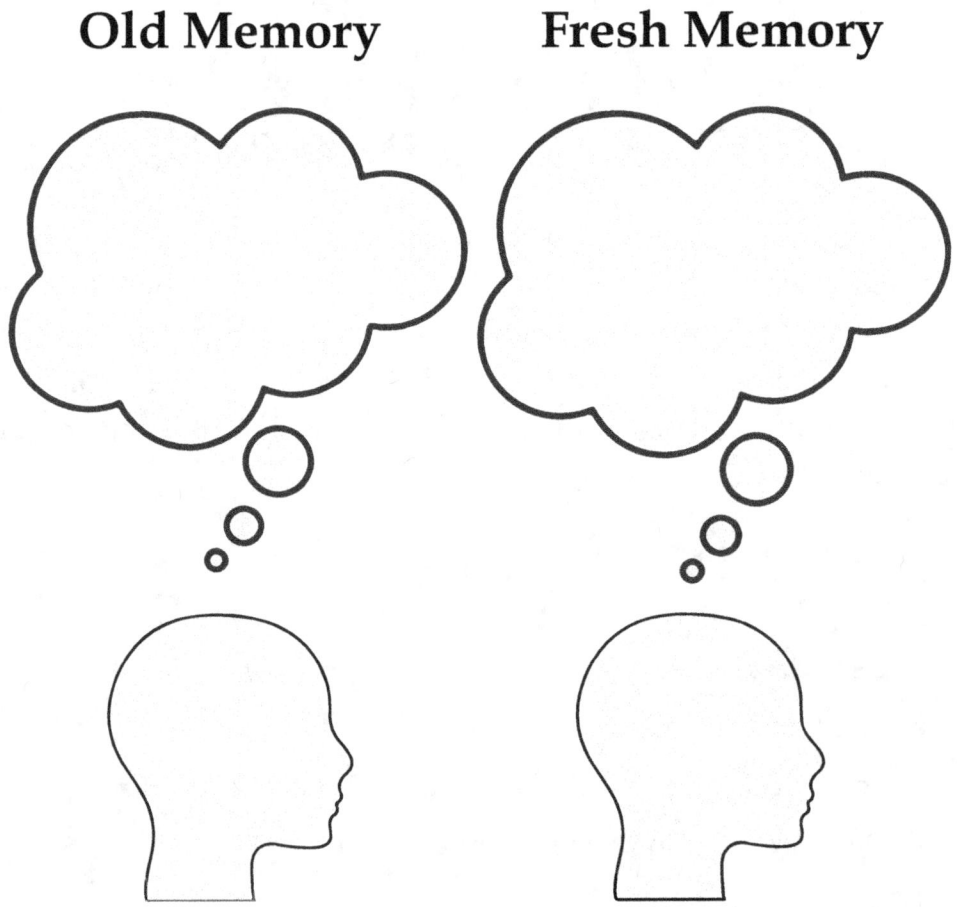

Concluding Remarks on Active Aging

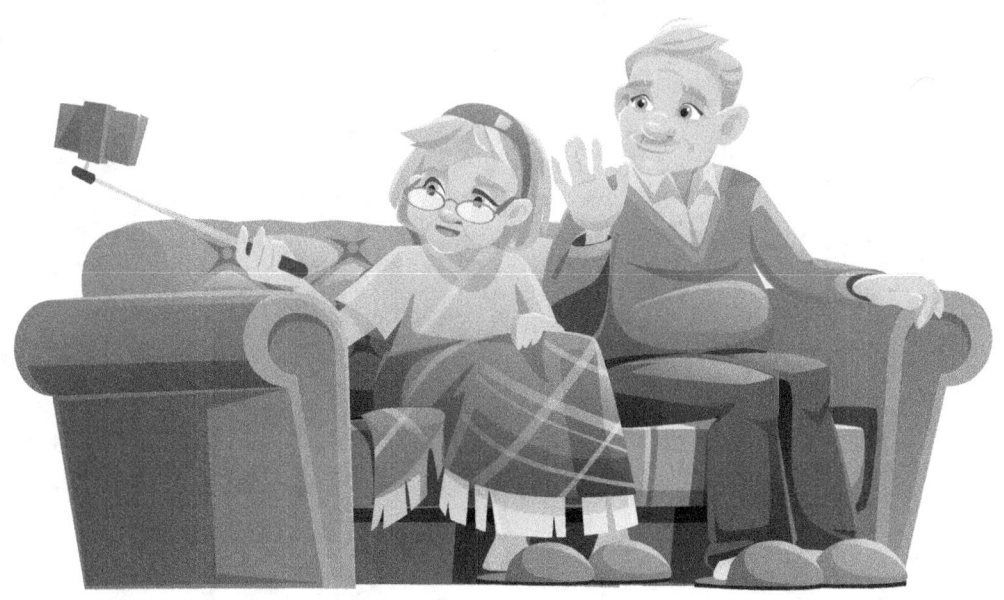

Who says seniors who have dementia can't enjoy fun and memory-stimulating games? Memory games have been proven to help exercise your mind, which is also necessary to boost your brain health. It's important to fully understand how essential it is to help prevent dementia from worsening.

As a living legend, you should always make your health a priority. Adding a little effort can help you achieve the quality of life you deserve. In this book, you have practiced quality and purpose-oriented worksheets designed to enhance your memory. Solving all these resources allows you to enjoy your life with dementia.

You can't reverse aging, but you can decide to age beautifully and productively.

Wishing you fun-filled golden years!

www.ingramcontent.com/pod-product-compliance
Lightning Source LLC
Chambersburg PA
CBHW081202290526
45796CB00010B/321